Current Practices in Sickle Cell Disease

Edited by Marwa Zakaria

Published in London, United Kingdom

Current Practices in Sickle Cell Disease
http://dx.doi.org/10.5772/intechopen.110970
Edited by Marwa Zakaria

Contributors
Abena Appiah-Kubi, Arushi Dhar, Banu Aygun, Elizabeth K. Fiorino, Elizabeth Mitchell, Grace K. Ababio, Lance Feld, La Nyka Christian-Weekes, Maria Teresa Santiago, Olivier Hermine, Oluwafemi Ajoyemi Ala, Rachel Rignault, Runyararo Mashingaidze Mano, Sampson Weytey, Slimane Allali, Thiago Trovati Maciel

First published in London, United Kingdom, 2024 by IntechOpen
IntechOpen is the global imprint of INTECHOPEN LIMITED, registered in England and Wales, registration number: 11086078, 167-169 Great Portland Street, London, W1W 5PF, United Kingdom

British Library Cataloguing-in-Publication Data
A catalogue record for this book is available from the British Library

Additional hard and PDF copies can be obtained from orders@intechopen.com

Current Practices in Sickle Cell Disease
Edited by Marwa Zakaria
p. cm.
Print ISBN 978-0-85466-920-2
Online ISBN 978-0-85466-919-6
eBook (PDF) ISBN 978-0-85466-921-9

Meet the editor

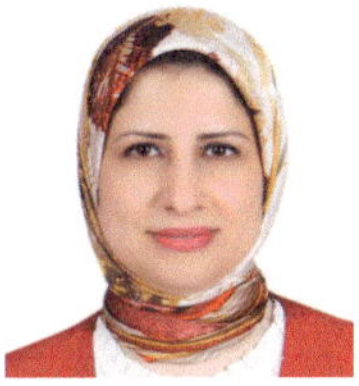

Dr. Zarakaria is a professor of pediatrics and pediatric hematology and oncology, Zagazig University, Egypt, and an active member of the International Society of Pediatric Oncology (SIOP), EHA, HAA, and ESPHO. Her professional training and workshops have included ICH GCP online training on May 2013 and February 2016; EHA master class 2015–2016 and EHA bite-size master class 2017–2018; and participation in many international and national pediatric and hematology conferences with EHA, SIOP, and Pan Arab Hematology Association. She has received training from the Wilkins-Barrack Society of Neurooncology (SNO), Marrakesh, Morocco, and completed the postgraduate training program in Pediatric Nutrition (School of Medicine, Boston University, 2017). She has completed international preceptorships including a Thalassemia Preceptorship (Beirut, Lebanon, September 7–9, 2015); International Hemophilia Preceptorship in Saint Luc Hospital, Brussels, Belgium; and International Hemophilia Preceptorship, December 12–15, 2022, Katharine Dormandy Hemophilia & Thrombosis Center, Royal Free London NHS Foundation Trust, London, UK. International awards include the award of SIOP for the year 2018 and the scholarship of EHA-HOPE Cairo for the years 2017 and. She has been a guest speaker at numerous international and national pediatric oncology and hematology meetings and has over 50 international publications. She is the academic editor of five online books and author of five online book chapters, as well as a reviewer in international and national journals (Medicine, IntechOpen publications, Spandidos publications, Frontiers in Pediatrics, Molecular Medicine Reports, International Journal of Infectious Diseases). She is an active member in the Sharkia Thalassemia Association, Egypt, and a member of the Egyptian National Guidelines Committee (NEGC) for evidence-based clinical practice. She has been a sub-investigator in many international hematology clinical trials.

Contents

Preface

Sickle cell disease is the most common monogenetic disease, with millions affected worldwide. Sickle cell disease is an inherited, multisystem disorder characterized by chronic hemolytic anemia, painful ischemic episodes of vaso-occlusion, and progressive organ failure. The vast majority of sickle cell disease births occur in sub-Saharan Africa. Due to the absence of newborn screening, 50% to 90% of these children will die undiagnosed in the first five years of their life. In contrast, in well-resourced countries, comprehensive care programs have increased life expectancy of sickle cell disease patients, with almost all infants surviving into adulthood. Therapeutic options for sickle cell disease patients are, however, still scarce. The only clinically available and notably safe disease-modifying treatment modalities are hydroxyurea and blood (exchange) transfusions. There are many pipelines of therapeutic options that will soon be available for those patients. Hematopoietic stem cell transplantation (HSCT) remains the only curative treatment option. Unfortunately, its use is limited by the lack of suitable donors and concerns about toxicity. Early results of gene therapy trials are promising and may form a potential alternative.

Marwa Zakaria
Professor of Pediatric Hematology and Oncology,
Faculty of Medicine,
Zagazig University,
Zagazig, Egypt

Chapter 1

Hemolysis and Innate Immunity Contribution to Sickle Cell Disease Pathophysiology

Thiago Trovati Maciel, Rachel Rignault, Slimane Allali and Olivier Hermine

Abstract

Sickle cell disease, recognized as the prevailing global monogenic ailment and a severe hemoglobin disorder, presents persistent challenges. Despite a well-established understanding of its genetic and molecular foundations, the pathophysiology remains partially elucidated, limiting therapeutic interventions. There's a growing acknowledgment of the involvement of innate immunity—monocytes, neutrophils, complement and mast cells—in promoting inflammation, adhesion, and pain in sickle cell disease. In this chapter, we explore the significant roles of these emerging key players in the pathophysiology of sickle cell disease. Emphasizing recent evidence, we underscore innovative therapeutic perspectives that could pave the way for more effective interventions in managing this complex disorder.

Keywords: sickle cell disease, hemolysis, inflammation, heme, hemoglobin, innate immunity

1. Introduction

Sickle cell disease (SCD) is a life-threatening genetic hemoglobin disorder, marked by persistent hemolytic anemia, recurrent painful vaso-occlusive events, and progressive damage to multiple organs. The global impact of SCD is significant, affecting millions of individuals worldwide, and projections suggest an increase to 400,000 neonates born annually with the condition by 2050 [1]. The disease's origins lie in a single nucleotide mutation of the β-globin gene, leading to the polymerization of abnormal deoxygenated hemoglobin S (HbS). This polymerization results in the obstruction of small vessels by sickle-shaped red blood cells (RBC) [2]. Despite this well-defined genetic and molecular basis, recent decades have unveiled a more intricate pathophysiology, extending beyond RBC involvement. This chapter seeks to delve into the intricate interplay with innate immunity, shedding light on the role of hemolysis in perpetuating chronic inflammation and influencing the diverse and often severe complications associated with SCD.

2. Understanding hemolysis in SCD

Hemolysis refers to the process where RBCs are destroyed and their contents released into the bloodstream. In the context of sickle cell disease, this process is exacerbated due to the abnormal shape and rigidity of the sickle cells, which makes them more prone to rupture. The HbS mutation, involving a single amino acid substitution in the β-globin chain, disrupts hemoglobin's structure and function, initiating a cascade of events. Under normal conditions, hemoglobin exists as isolated units within RBCs when they are oxygenated. However, when HbS releases oxygen in peripheral tissues, the molecules tend to stick together and form long chains or polymers. These rigid polymers distort the cell, causing it to bend out of shape. The resulting sickled RBCs are less flexible and more prone to deformation, leading to a shorter lifespan when compared to normal RBCs and impairing their ability to flow smoothly through blood vessels. These abnormal cells can get stuck, leading to vaso-occlusion and tissue damage [3].

SCD is characterized by chronic hemolysis, with roughly 66% occurring extravascularly and 33% intra-vascularly [4]. This cellular breakdown plays a critical role in the pathological mechanisms and diverse clinical complications associated with SCD. Notably, both extravascular and intravascular hemolysis contribute to vaso-occlusive pain crisis and various other health problems experienced by individuals with SCD.

2.1 Extravascular hemolysis

Extravascular hemolysis in SCD is an intricate physiological process instigated by the distinctive polymerization of HbS within RBCs. This phenomenon holds profound consequences, precipitating marked alterations in RBC integrity and viability [5]. Macrophages play a pivotal role in the recognition and subsequent phagocytosis of these aberrant RBCs.

The process of macrophage phagocytosis, central to extravascular hemolysis, unfolds prominently in the spleen and liver within the reticuloendothelial system. Macrophages play a crucial role in protecting the body by clearing the contents of altered RBCs. This process, known as erythrophagocytosis, involves the phagocytosis of modified RBCs by macrophages, preventing the release of inflammatory hemoglobin and heme into the extracellular space [6]. Macrophages, particularly those in the splenic red pulp, are strategically located near RBCs and express specific molecules like SIRP-α. These molecules enable macrophages to identify and phagocytize damaged or senescent RBCs, as they interact with CD47 on the surface of healthy RBCs, providing an inhibitory signal [7]. Erythrophagocytosis leads to increased intracellular heme concentrations in macrophages, transforming them into erythrophagocytes for iron recycling. Simultaneously, antioxidative and anti-inflammatory pathways are activated to protect against hemolytic stress. This intricate process underscores the vital role of macrophages in maintaining homeostasis by efficiently clearing altered RBCs and managing their contents.

Splenic sequestration involves the critical trapping and retention of sickled RBCs. Splenic sequestration crises pose life-threatening risks attributable to acute anemia and organ enlargement [8]. The spleen is particularly susceptible to damage in SCD due to its open microcirculation, creating an environment conducive to in vivo deoxygenation and subsequent sickling of RBCs. This sickling process increases the expression of adhesion molecules and activates proteins that are typically dormant, leading to the adherence of RBCs to the spleen matrix or macrophages [9]. Additionally, non-receptor mechanisms, such as the pro-adhesive roles of red cell sulphated glycolipids and phosphatidyl serine, contribute to enhanced clearance through phagocytosis, contributing to the shortened lifespan of sickle RBCs. The impaired deformability of sickled RBCs further facilitates their trapping upstream by narrow inter-endothelial slits [8]. At the molecular level, the intricacies of splenic sequestration involve membrane rigidity. Oxidative damage profoundly impacts actin filaments, inducing a slow dissociation of the spectrin-actin-4.1 complex [10]. This rigidity significantly impedes the ability of sickled RBCs to regain their normal discoid shape upon exposure to atmospheric oxygen.

Transitioning beyond the spleen, hepatic clearance in SCD substantively contributes to liver injury through mechanisms such as vaso-occlusion, intense hemolysis, and sterile inflammation. Approximately 10–40% of SCD patients experience hepatic dysfunction, a statistic corroborated by comprehensive clinical studies and patient cohorts [11]. Acute sickle hepatic sequestration is characterized by hepatomegaly resulting from the sequestration of sickled erythrocytes in the hepatic vasculature and spleen, accompanied by acute anemia. This condition shares clinical symptoms with acute sickle hepatic crisis, presenting with significant organ enlargement and a rapid decrease in hemoglobin levels, potentially leading to hypovolemic shock. It is crucial to note that acute sickle intrahepatic cholestasis, a severe variant of sickle hepatopathy, has a high mortality rate and is rare, primarily affecting individuals with homozygous HbSS genotypes. Clinical manifestations of this condition include transaminase elevations, hyperbilirubinemia, severe jaundice, renal failure, and coagulopathy. The pathophysiology involves sickling of erythrocytes within sinusoids, resulting in ischemia, hepatocyte injury, hepatocyte ballooning, and canalicular cholestasis. Acute sickle intrahepatic cholestasis demands careful attention due to its severe nature and potential life-threatening complications [12].

These insights into the sophisticated interplay of molecular events underscore the complexity of extravascular hemolysis in SCD, necessitating ongoing scientific inquiry for a comprehensive understanding and the development of effective therapeutic strategies.

2.2 Intravascular hemolysis

In the pathophysiology of SCD, intravascular hemolysis emerges as a pivotal process wherein RBCs succumb to destruction within the blood vessels, resulting in the release of cellular contents, notably hemoglobin and heme, into the bloodstream [13, 14]. The intricate mechanisms governing the breakdown of sickled RBCs within the bloodstream encompass several key forces, each contributing to the overall hemolytic cascade.

As sickled cells traverse the narrow microvasculature, they experience significant shear stress. This mechanical stress, particularly accentuated in hypoxic conditions, plays a direct role in rupturing the membranes of sickled RBCs, thereby triggering the process of hemolysis. The nuances of shear stress-induced hemolysis have been elucidated through advanced imaging techniques, such as microfluidic models and intravital microscopy, providing insights into the dynamic interplay between sickled RBCs and vascular shear forces [15].

The sickling phenomenon also disrupts the normal metabolism of RBCs, leading to an upsurge in the production of reactive oxygen species (ROS). These highly reactive molecules induce significant damage to cellular components, encompassing RBC membranes and hemoglobin, thereby intensifying the hemolytic process. In addition, the accumulation of oxidative injury might also contribute to exposure of phosphatidylserine, and ultimately, RBC cell death and phagocytosis [16]. Scientific studies employing mass spectrometry and advanced imaging technologies have allowed for a detailed exploration of the molecular pathways involved in sickle cell-induced oxidative stress and its impact on hemolysis.

Despite the plethora of pathways contributing to ROS generation in SCD, patients typically exhibit compensated oxidative stress levels during steady states. However, this delicate balance between ROS production and antioxidants becomes disrupted during crises, characterized by excessive ROS generation, diminished antioxidant levels, or a combination of both [17]. Studies investigating antioxidant levels in SCD patients have yielded divergent outcomes, with certain studies reporting diminished activity of antioxidant enzymes such as glutathione peroxidase, superoxide dismutase and catalase, while others indicate elevated levels [18, 19]. These discrepancies may be attributed to variations in disease severity, encompassing factors such as hemolysis, lipid peroxidation, vaso-occlusive crisis, acute splenic sequestration, and pulmonary hypertension observed in these patients [20]. Regardless of the detected levels, the cumulative antioxidant capacity in SCD patients remains inadequate to counterbalance excess ROS, thereby perpetuating oxidative stress [21].

The presence of extracellular hemoglobin and heme in the bloodstream, insufficiently neutralized by haptoglobin and hemopexin, contributes significantly to oxidative stress [22]. It is noteworthy that haptoglobin exhibits limited recyclability, and its levels can be depleted following extensive hemolysis, consequently allowing for the accumulation of free hemoglobin. Within the plasma milieu, liberated hemoglobin is prone to oxidation, resulting in the formation of higher hemoglobin iron oxidation states, such as methemoglobin (FeIII) and ferryl-hemoglobin (FeIV). These non-functional hemoglobin forms exhibit an inability to bind molecular oxygen and readily release associated heme groups [23]. The released heme, often termed free heme, exhibits a high hydrophobicity, leading it to loosely bind to plasma acceptor proteins and lipids, rather than existing in its fully free form. In this loosely bound state, termed labile heme, it retains redox activity, readily exchanging with other proteins.

Hemoglobin can react with hydrogen peroxide, leading to the formation of hydroxyl free radicals and methemoglobin, especially when released into plasma and dissociated into dimers. During the process of intravascular hemolysis, the hemoglobin released from lysed cells exhibits a pronounced affinity for nitric oxide (NO), a potent vasodilator. This avid binding results in NO depletion, fostering vasoconstriction, reduced blood flow, and further damage to RBCs, thereby establishing a self-perpetuating cycle of hemolysis. This accelerated NO consumption significantly reduces NO bioavailability in individuals with SCD [24]. Further supporting this proposition, Gladwin et al. [25] observed a nullification of blood flow responses to the NO donor sodium nitroprusside in patients with the highest plasma heme levels. This observation implies that NO scavenging or inactivation, mediated by heightened plasma hemoglobin levels, significantly contributes to impaired vascular responsiveness. Recent studies have linked microvascular regulation impairment in SCD children to peroxynitrite and oxidative stress markers [26].

Upon release from hemoglobin, labile heme initially binds to albumin, the predominant protein in plasma. Subsequently, it is transferred to hemopexin, the most effective heme-binding protein, even though its presence in plasma at lower concentrations [27]. The resultant hemopexin-heme complexes undergo recognition and clearance from circulation through the binding to and internalization by the scavenger receptor CD91 on hepatocytes and macrophages. This process is succeeded by heme catabolism, wherein heme is broken down by the heme-oxygenase (HO-1) system, facilitating ferrous iron recycling by ferritin [28].

In instances of excessive hemolysis, the saturation and depletion of heme scavenging proteins lead to the accumulation of free heme in the plasma. The formation of low-affinity complexes between free heme and plasma proteins fails to effectively restrain its redox activity [29]. Free heme, characterized by its pro-oxidant and pro-inflammatory potential, poses a cytotoxic threat to cells. Its extreme hydrophobicity facilitates easy penetration into the phospholipid bilayer and intercalation into lipid membranes, exacerbating heme toxicity. Consequently, the cytotoxicity of heme contributes to the activation of the innate immune response, cytokine release, and tissue damage, underscoring the multifaceted consequences of intravascular hemolysis in sickle cell disease [30].

2.3 Hemolysis-specific complications in SCD

Hemoglobin liberated during intravascular hemolysis undergoes a dynamic fate within the circulatory system. Its scavenging by haptoglobin, followed by complex formation with CD163 (hemoglobin scavenger receptor) on macrophages and subsequent phagocytosis and degradation, depletes plasma haptoglobin. The accumulation of cell-free plasma hemoglobin becomes evident only when the hemolytic rate surpasses the scavenging capacity of plasma haptoglobin [14]. This accumulated hemoglobin engages in a stoichiometric reaction with NO, effectively inactivating it through a nearly diffusion-limited process, thereby perpetuating the intricate interplay between intravascular hemolysis and NO dynamics in the context of SCD. One of the primary complications linked to NO scavenging and hemolysis in SCD is pulmonary hypertension, a condition characterized by high blood pressure in the arteries that supply blood to the lungs. In SCD, decreased bioavailability of NO, which act as a potent vasodilator, leads to vasoconstriction. This vasoconstriction can increase the pressure in the pulmonary arteries, leading to pulmonary hypertension [31]. Studies have shown that pulmonary hypertension is a significant predictor of mortality in adults with SCD.

Another complication specifically linked to hemolysis in SCD is leg ulcers. Leg ulcers are open sores that develop on the skin, usually on the lower legs. In SCD, these ulcers are believed to occur due to a combination of factors including impaired blood flow due to vaso-occlusion, local hypoxia, and inflammation. The hemolysis-associated reduction in NO bioavailability can further exacerbate these factors, leading to the development of leg ulcers [32]. Hemolysis in SCD can also lead to other complications such as renal dysfunction and stroke. The free hemoglobin and other cell-free heme proteins released during hemolysis can cause oxidative stress and inflammation, damaging various organs including the kidneys [13]. Similarly, the reduction in NO bioavailability can impair cerebral blood flow, increasing the risk of stroke.

3. Contribution of innate immune cells to the pathophysiology of SCD

3.1 Monocytes and macrophages

Monocytes emerge as crucial players in the intricate pathophysiology of SCD. Notably, monocytosis is a prevailing feature in SCD, exhibiting positive correlation with hemolysis markers and an inverse relationship with hemoglobin levels [33]. Monocyte count in SCD children under hydroxyurea treatment is lower, hinting at potential positive impacts of the therapy [34]. In vitro studies unveil the heightened oxidative stress induced by SCD patients' RBC on cultured human umbilical vein endothelial cells, escalating trans-endothelial migration of monocytes [35].

Monocytes from SCD patients exhibit increased CD11b surface expression, along with heightened production of proinflammatory cytokines IL-1β and TNF-α, diverging from the subdued state of healthy control monocytes [36]. NADPH oxidase components' upregulation results in increased superoxide anion production by SCD monocytes [37]. Furthermore, circulating tissue factor-positive monocytes spike in numbers, contributing to observed coagulation abnormalities in SCD patients. The expression of tissue factor on monocytes correlates positively with pain rate, C-reactive protein levels, and reticulocyte percentage, while inversely linked to hemoglobin concentration. This hints at hemolysis and inflammation influencing SCD monocyte activation [38].

Activated monocytes from SCD patients also play a pivotal role in endothelial cell activation via the nuclear factor (NF)-κB pathway. This activation leads to elevated expression of endothelial adhesion molecules such as E-selectin, intracellular adhesion molecule 1 (ICAM-1), and vascular cell adhesion molecule 1 (VCAM-1) [36]. IL-1β and TNF-α, produced by SCD monocytes, mediate endothelial activation, as confirmed by neutralizing antibodies targeting these cytokines. In transgenic sickle mice, the monocyte–TNF-α–endothelial activation axis gains prominence, with TNF-α blockers showing more comprehensive benefits than IL-1β blockers [39].

Hypoxemia emerges as a suspected player in monocyte activation, with nocturnal oxygen saturation correlating inversely with CD11b expression in SCD children [40]. Platelet-monocyte aggregates increase in SCD patients, potentially pointing to platelet-induced monocyte activation [41]. Moreover, interactions with activated sickle RBC, circulating platelet-monocyte aggregates, and plasma fibronectin bridge formation further highlight the intricate network inducing monocyte activation [42].

Recent revelations spotlight a distinctive subset of patrolling monocytes expressing high levels of HO-1 in SCD patients [43]. These cells display remarkable abilities to scavenge cellular debris from damaged vascular endothelium, especially when exposed to heme. In mice, the absence of patrolling monocytes exacerbates vascular stasis in the presence of sickle RBC, hinting at their protective role against vaso-occlusive crisis. Patrolling monocytes demonstrate enhanced survival by upregulating HO-1, countering the cytotoxic effects of RBC-engulfed material. Further exploration is warranted to unveil the full extent of their potential in removing other blood cells attached to the endothelium during vaso-occlusive crisis.

In SCD, liver macrophages undergo polarization towards an M1 pro-inflammatory phenotype, characterized by heightened TNF-α and IL-6 expression. This shift may contribute to liver damage, triggering monocyte recruitment, cytokine overproduction, hepatocyte apoptosis, and fibrosis [44]. Heme, a key player in this process, induces the phenotypic switch in macrophages. IL-1β, originating from macrophages and activated by heme through the NLRP3 inflammasome, emerges as a potential contributor to SCD pathogenesis. Hemopexin administration attenuates the pro-inflammatory status of liver macrophages, offering insights into therapeutic avenues [45].

As the role of monocytes and macrophages in SCD unfolds, the landscape becomes more complex, offering new avenues for understanding and potentially mitigating the disease's impact.

3.2 Neutrophils

Neutrophils emerge as pivotal contributors to the intricate pathophysiology of SCD. In steady-state SCD, the absolute neutrophil count is notably higher than in healthy controls, correlating positively with disease severity [46]. Elevated leukocyte count in SCD patients serves as a risk factor for various complications, including early mortality, acute chest syndrome, hemorrhagic stroke, and sickle nephropathy. Conversely, decreased neutrophil count, induced by hydroxyurea treatment, aligns with potential positive effects on the SCD phenotype, suggesting a delicate balance in managing neutrophil levels [47]. SCD patients exhibit an activated state of neutrophils, characterized by increased adhesive properties, particularly accentuated during vaso-occlusive crisis. Clinical manifestations in SCD are associated with the expression of adhesion molecules on neutrophils. Hydroxyurea shows potential benefits by suppressing neutrophil activation and rectifying dysregulated adhesion marker expression [48]. Neutrophil adhesion to activated endothelium involves various mediators, including endothelin-1. Elevated plasma levels of endothelin-1 in SCD patients upregulate TNF-α–induced Mac-1 expression on neutrophils. Targeting endothelin receptors, especially endothelin B receptor, attenuates neutrophil recruitment, suggesting therapeutic potential [49].

Intravital microscopy in SCD mice reveals heightened neutrophil adhesion not only to endothelium but also to sickle RBC in postcapillary venules [50]. E-selectin induces a secondary wave of signals leading to the clustering of activated macrophage-1 antigen (Mac-1) on adherent neutrophils, facilitating the capture of sickle RBC and platelets. Targeting E-selectin or Mac-1 in mice prevents neutrophil–RBC and neutrophil–platelet interactions, enhancing blood flow and mouse survival [51]. Clinical trials showcase promising results with selectin antagonists. Rivipansel, a pan-selectin antagonist, and crizanlizumab, specifically targeting P-selectin, demonstrate efficacy in reducing vaso-occlusive events in SCD patients [52, 53]. Rivipansel exhibits improved blood flow and reduced opioid analgesic use. Crizanlizumab significantly reduces the median rate of vaso-occlusive crisis per year, leading to its approval by the US Food and Drug Administration.

SCD patients exhibit high proportions of aged neutrophils, positively correlated with endothelial adhesion, Mac-1 expression, and neutrophil extracellular trap (NET) formation [54]. Neutrophil aging appears linked to microbiota via TLR/Myd88 signaling, offering insights into the impact of prophylactic antibiotic treatment. Elevated plasma heme levels during vaso-occlusive crisis promote NET formation, suggesting their involvement in acute chest syndrome pathogenesis [55]. Heme-induced NETs may also contribute to susceptibility to infections by impairing neutrophils' bactericidal capabilities.

The role of neutrophils in SCD spans a multifaceted landscape, from adhesive interactions to intricate signaling pathways. Therapeutic strategies targeting neutrophil dynamics show promise but demand further exploration to decipher their full potential in mitigating the complex pathophysiology of SCD. As research advances, the intricate dance between neutrophils, endothelium, and other blood components becomes clearer, offering hope for more effective interventions in the future.

3.3 Mast cells

Growing evidence implicates mast cells in SCD pathophysiology, particularly in chronic pain resembling mastocytosis and clinical signs of mast cell activation syndrome [56]. Plasma levels of mast cell mediators, including histamine and substance P, are elevated in steady-state, escalating during vaso-occlusive crisis [57, 58]. Histamine, negatively correlated with HbF levels, may contribute to SCD pathogenesis by promoting adhesion of sickle RBC. Substance P, acting as a primary pain neurotransmitter, further intertwines with mast cell activation, forming a cycle of activation and release.

Inhibition of mast cells, achieved through mast-cell stabilizers like cromolyn or c-kit/tyrosine kinase inhibitor imatinib, proves effective in reducing substance

P and tryptase levels, systemic inflammation, neurogenic inflammation, and hyperalgesia in SCD mice [59]. Results, replicated in transgenic SCD mice lacking mast cells, underline the therapeutic potential. Pre-clinical and clinical evidence with imatinib, demonstrating resolution of vaso-occlusive crisis [60, 61], prompts consideration for a clinical trial with c-kit/tyrosine kinase inhibitors in SCD patients.

In SCD mice, high-affinity opioid nociception receptor agonist AT-200, inhibiting substance P release from sensory nerve endings, exhibits superior antinociceptive effects compared to morphine. Morphine, commonly used for vaso-occlusive crisis in SCD patients, stimulates substance P release from mast cells, exacerbating neurogenic inflammation [59]. Human mast-cell degranulation induced by morphine through MAS-related G-protein-coupled receptor X2 (MRGPRX2) raises concerns about the drug's impact.

Mast cells have recently emerged as key players of SCD pathophysiology, offering potential therapeutic targets. Understanding their roles in inflammation, organ damage, and pain opens avenues for precise interventions. The intricate interplay between mast cells and various molecular mediators demands further exploration for comprehensive management of SCD complications. As research advances, these cellular players may hold the key to unraveling the complexities of SCD and devising more effective treatment strategies.

3.4 Complement

Compelling evidence for complement activation in SCD is rooted in the consistent elevation of distinct complement activation fragments across diverse SCD patient cohorts, both during vaso-occlusive crisis and at baseline. Notably, elevated Bb levels during vaso-occlusive crisis highlight the involvement of the alternative [62]. Furthermore, the presence of complexes formed by C3 and properdin, indicative of alternative pathway activation, is consistently elevated. Specific indicators, such as increased C3a levels (with no parallel rise in C4d), underscore predominant alternative pathway activation during vaso-occlusive crisis, reinforcing the multifaceted nature of complement involvement [62].

Evidence for complement activation extends to the surface of SCD RBCs, further substantiating alternative pathway activation. Increased C3d-bearing RBCs at steady state and a surge during vaso-occlusive crisis indicate active complement involvement [63]. In vitro models demonstrate specific alternative pathway activation in the presence of SCD RBCs, progressing to terminal pathway activation, heightening susceptibility to C5b-9-mediated lysis [64]. Moreover, incubation of SCD RBCs with normal human serum accentuates sC5b-9 release, emphasizing the distinct nature of complement dynamics in SCD [65].

Detection of complement products within SCD tissues offers a macroscopic dimension to complement activation. Renal involvement in SCD nephropathy is underscored by C3c and C9 deposition in the kidney [66]. Additionally, C5b-9, the final complement product, is observed in small skin vessels, providing evidence for intra-microvascular complement system activation [67]. Studies from HbSS mice underscores complement activation not only intravascularly, as evidenced by increased factor B cleavage during vaso-occlusive crisis, but also within tissues. Elevated C3 activation fragments and C5b-9 deposits in tissues like kidneys, livers, and lungs highlight the systemic complement involvement, especially post-hypoxia/reoxygenation, a vaso-occlusive crisis model used in vivo [66].

Extracellular release of hemoglobin and cell-free heme, hallmark features of SCD hemolysis, emerges as a major trigger for complement activation. Heme, with its broad protein-binding capacity, modulates the activity of several complement proteins. It influences classical pathway activation by altering C1q activity while promoting alternative pathway activation and amplification through interactions with C3 and its fragments [68].

The mounting evidence points unequivocally to complement activation in SCD patients, spanning alternative and terminal pathways, systemic compartments, RBC surfaces, and tissues. The intricate dynamics at play underscore the need for a comprehensive understanding of complement activation mechanisms in SCD. As research progresses, insights into these complexities could pave the way for targeted interventions aimed at modulating complement activation for improved outcomes in SCD patients.

4. Impact of hemolysis on SCD inflammation

Hemolysis releases danger-associated molecular patterns like free-heme and free-hemoglobin, triggering the activation of innate immune cells, primarily monocytes and macrophages. These activated cells churn out a plethora of pro-inflammatory cytokines, chemokines, and adhesion molecules, creating a chronic inflammatory milieu that underpins various SCD complications.

4.1 Inflammatory cascades triggered by hemolysis

In individuals diagnosed with SCD, there is an observed elevation of proinflammatory cytokines, such as TNF- α, IL-6 and IL-1β, induced by NF-κB signaling. These elevated levels are present both at baseline and during vaso-occlusive crisis. The heightened cytokine levels contribute to the activation of inflammatory cells, causing damage to endothelial cells, and ultimately exacerbating vaso-occlusion (**Figure 1**) [36].

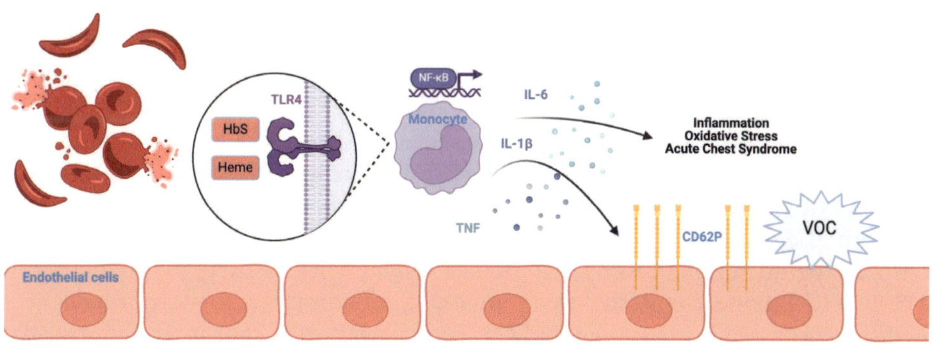

Figure 1.
Proposed mechanism of inflammatory cascades triggered by hemolysis in SCD, involving heme, HbS, TLR4, and NF-kB activation. Intravascular hemolysis contributes to elevated levels of free heme and endothelial cells activation during vaso-occlusive events [69] and initiate the NLRP3 inflammasome pathway, leading to IL-1β release [70] and P-selectin (CD62P) externalization. Heme activates TLR4 through MD-2 binding [71, 72], inducing NF-κB activation and consequently production of inflammatory cytokines IL-6 and TNF-α. Chronic hemolysis in SCD results in elevated plasma heme, contributing to vaso-occlusion and lung injury, with heme-induced TLR4 activation being a primary driver. The release of free HbS in SCD triggers monocyte activation and cytokine production [73]. Inhibiting TLR4 reduces vaso-occlusive crisis and protects against heme-mediated acute lung injury in mouse models, highlighting the significance of this HbS/heme activation through TLR4 signaling in regulating inflammation in SCD.

Additionally, recent findings highlight increased levels of type 1 interferons (IFN-α/β) in SCD patients, with potential implications during RBC transfusion and viral infections [74]. Despite these known associations, there is a gap in understanding the specific triggers for cytokine production in SCD.

4.2 Hemolysis, innate immunity and acute chest syndrome

Acute chest syndrome (ACS), a severe and potentially life-threatening form of acute lung injury in SCD, is characterized by fever, respiratory symptoms, and a new pulmonary infiltrate on chest radiograph [75]. Despite being a major contributor to morbidity and premature death in SCD patients, the underlying mechanisms of ACS remain incompletely understood, limiting therapeutic options. Various factors, including infection, hypoventilation during vaso-occlusive crisis, fat embolism, and thromboembolism, may contribute to ACS development. In cases of severe ACS with acute respiratory failure, the pathogenesis remains unclear. Ischemia/reperfusion and hemolysis-induced inflammation are suggested factors, potentially mediated by the activation of lung endothelium and innate immune cells [55].

The Cooperative Study of Sickle Cell Disease identified severe acute hemolysis as the sole predictor of sudden death due to ACS [76]. Ghosh et al. [55] reported in a mice model of SCD a mechanism of acute lung injury involving extracellular hemin that may have important ramifications for the diagnosis, prevention, and treatment of ACS. In this study, TLR4 expressed in the vessel wall was found to be essential for the pathogenesis of this murine model of acute lung injury, with therapeutic roles for targeting the acute adverse effects of plasma free heme with hemopexin and by TLR4 blockade. Thus, a vascular inflammatory response to excess extracellular hemin may play a central role in the pathogenesis of ACS.

IL-6 emerges as a central proinflammatory cytokine, intricately woven into the fabric of cellular communication across various tissues. With a widespread cellular origin including macrophages, neutrophils, endothelial and smooth muscle cells, cardiomyocytes, and fibroblasts, IL-6 plays a pivotal role in diverse biological functions, spanning hematopoiesis, oncogenesis, B cell differentiation, induction of acute phase proteins, and immune regulation [77].

Recent findings indicate a potential link between massive production of IL-6 in the lungs and ACS pathophysiology, independent of systemic inflammation. High sputum IL-6 levels (>6000 pg/mL) were associated with severe ACS forms, indicating its potential as a marker of severity [78]. In a prospective study, C-reactive protein (CRP) and sputum IL-6 levels were identified as biological markers associated with ACS occurrence during vaso-occlusive crisis. The combination of sputum IL-6 > 150 pg/mL and/or CRP >150 mg/L showed higher sensitivity for predicting ACS than CRP alone, suggesting that pulmonary inflammation may occur independently of systemic inflammation [79]. Early detection of sputum IL-6 during vaso-occlusive crisis may enable preventive treatment strategies, such as anti-human IL-6 receptor monoclonal antibody (e.g., tocilizumab) as recently reported in a case of severe ACS in a child with SCD and high IL-6 levels in endotracheal and pleural fluids [80].

Understanding the role of hemolysis in ACS is crucial for developing targeted therapeutic strategies. Interventions aimed at mitigating hemolysis-related processes, such as anti-inflammatory agents, antioxidants, and agents that preserve nitric oxide bioavailability, may hold promise in preventing and managing ACS in individuals with SCD. Moreover, ongoing research continues to unravel the intricate connections between hemolysis and ACS, providing opportunities for improved clinical management and outcomes.

4.3 Protective aspects of immune response

Within the realm of protective mechanisms, the immune response to hemolysis in SCD orchestrates a multifaceted defense strategy. Firstly, the complement system and macrophages act collaboratively to identify and eliminate senescent or hemolyzed RBCs, mitigating the accumulation of potentially harmful molecules within the circulation. This orchestrated clearance mechanism serves as a critical bulwark against the detrimental effects of unchecked hemolysis.

Additionally, the innate immune system's rapid and effective response against invading pathogens plays a pivotal role in averting infections that could trigger vaso-occlusive crisis in SCD. Pro-inflammatory cytokines, chemokines, and type I interferons orchestrate the activation and recruitment of immune cells, including macrophages, neutrophils, and natural killer (NK) cells. These immune effectors engage in phagocytosis, destruction, or secretion of antimicrobial substances, fortifying the host's defense against potential pathogens.

Furthermore, the immune response induces adaptive immunity, generating specific and enduring defenses against pathogens. Pattern recognition receptors (PRRs) stimulate the maturation and migration of dendritic cells, which, in turn, present antigens to T and B cells, activating and differentiating them. The complement system enhances this process by binding to complement receptors on B cells and follicular dendritic cells, bolstering the antibody response.

4.4 Deleterious consequences of immune response

Conversely, the immune response to hemolysis in SCD unveils a dark side marked by harmful consequences. Excessive or prolonged activation of the innate immune system sparks chronic inflammation and tissue injury, evident through the induction of adhesion molecules (e.g., VCAM-1, ICAM-1, and E-selectin) on the endothelium. These molecules facilitate the attachment and infiltration of leukocytes into tissues, releasing reactive oxygen and nitrogen species, proteases, and metalloproteinases that contribute to endothelial and surrounding cell damage.

Additionally, the immune response can trigger autoimmune and alloimmune reactions in SCD. Exposure of RBC antigens prompts the production of autoantibodies or alloantibodies, targeting and destroying the patient's own RBCs or transfused donor RBCs. This culminates in conditions such as hemolytic anemia, hemolytic transfusion reactions, or hyperhemolysis syndrome, exacerbating the clinical outcomes of SCD.

Moreover, impaired NO bioavailability due to hemolysis interferes with the NO signaling pathway, resulting in a dysregulated immune response. The reduced NO bioavailability leads to heightened inflammation and diminished regulation, as NO normally inhibits T cell activation and proliferation, influences the function of Th1 and Th17 cells, modulates antigen-presenting cells, and regulates the production of pro-inflammatory cytokines.

In conclusion, hemolysis in SCD shapes innate immune responses by activating PRRs, modulating the complement system, and impairing NO bioavailability. These responses, inherently dual in nature, harbor the potential for both beneficial and detrimental effects on disease outcomes. The intricate balance between host defense and tissue damage, autoimmunity and allo-immunity, as well as inflammation and regulation, remains pivotal. A comprehensive understanding of the mechanisms and consequences of the immune response to hemolysis in SCD holds promise for unveiling novel insights and therapeutic interventions.

5. Therapeutic strategies targeting hemolysis and innate immunity

(See **Table 1**)

Therapeutic Strategy	Description	Perspectives and Limitations
Hydroxyurea	Induces fetal hemoglobin, reducing HbS polymerization and subsequent hemolysis.	Ongoing exploration across diverse patient populations for optimized impact and long-term safety.
Nucleic Acid Therapeutics	Explore antisense oligonucleotides and gene silencing for suppressing HbS or enhancing HbF.	Ongoing research refines mechanisms and offers alternatives to gene therapy.
Small Molecules	Target specific pathways to prevent sickling and hemolysis without inducing HbF, facilitating more focused pharmacological interventions.	Cost effective approaches to cover large amount of patients world-wide.
Corticosteroids	Provide transient relief during acute complications.	Challenges with prolonged use due to notable side effects, emphasizing the need for refined therapeutic strategies.
IL-1β Inhibitors	Show promise in alleviating pain and reducing inflammatory markers.	Continued research is crucial for understanding long-term efficacy and safety.
IL-6 Inhibitors	Under investigation for managing chronic inflammation and improving lung function in SCD.	Explore their impact on specific inflammatory pathways for therapeutic optimization.
Specific Toll-like Receptor Antagonists	Target receptors like TLR4 to minimize side effects in anti-inflammatory interventions.	Research is necessary to overcome risk of infection on SCD patients.
JAK Inhibitors	Offer broader anti-inflammatory activity by suppressing cytokine receptor signaling pathways.	Pre-clinical research is needed to understand their role in modulating cytokine networks and long-term implications.
Precision Medicine	Tailor therapies based on individual inflammatory profiles, aiming for maximum efficacy with minimal side effects.	Integration of advanced technologies and comprehensive patient profiling will be pivotal for this approach.
Stem Cell Therapy	Based on mesenchymal stem cells with immunomodulatory properties to mitigate inflammation and promote tissue repair in SCD.	Research is necessary to explore mechanisms, optimal sources, and long-term effects for therapeutic development.
Nutritional Interventions	Optimize dietary intake and address micronutrient deficiencies to reduce oxidative stress and support immune function.	Evaluation of their impact on redox homeostasis for comprehensive disease management is necessary.

Table 1.
Overview of therapeutic strategies for SCD. Summary of various therapeutic strategies for managing SCD, detailing their mechanisms, perspectives, and limitations. These strategies range from pharmacological interventions such as hydroxyurea and small molecules, to advanced approaches like nucleic acid therapeutics, stem cell therapy, and precision medicine. Each strategy's potential benefits are weighed against ongoing research requirements and challenges to optimize their impact on diverse patient populations.

6. Conclusion: a path towards a brighter future

While dealing with the complexity of SCD is challenging, there's hope for improved outcomes through advancing therapies. By focusing on reducing hemolysis, adjusting the body's natural defense mechanisms, and tailoring treatments to each individual, we will not just manage problems one by one but create a future where SCD has much less impact. Achieving this optimistic vision relies on continuous research to better understand SCD, leading to improved care and quality of live for those affected.

Author details

Thiago Trovati Maciel[1*], Rachel Rignault[1], Slimane Allali[2] and Olivier Hermine[3]

1 Imagine Institute, University Paris Cité, Paris, France

2 Department of General Paediatrics and Paediatric Infectious Diseases, Sickle Cell Centre, Assistance Publique - Hôpitaux de Paris (AP-HP), Necker-Enfants Malades Hospital, Imagine Institute, Université Paris Cité, Paris, France

3 Department of Hematology, Necker-Enfants Malades Hospital, AP-HP, Imagine Institute, Université Paris Cité, Paris, France

*Address all correspondence to: thiago.trovati@inserm.fr

References

[1] Piel FB, Hay SI, Gupta S, Weatherall DJ, Williams TN. Global burden of sickle cell anaemia in children under five, 2010-2050: Modelling based on demographics, excess mortality, and interventions. PLoS Medicine. 2013;**10**(7):e1001484. DOI: 10.1371/journal.pmed.1001484

[2] Sundd P, Gladwin MT, Novelli EM. Pathophysiology of sickle cell disease. Annual Review of Pathology. 2019;**14**:263-292. DOI: 10.1146/annurev-pathmechdis-012418-012838

[3] Eaton WA, Bunn HF. Treating sickle cell disease by targeting HbS polymerization. Blood. 2017;**129**(20):2719-2726. DOI: 10.1182/blood-2017-02-765891

[4] Bensinger TA, Gillette PN. Hemolysis in sickle cell disease. Archives of Internal Medicine. 1974;**133**(4):624-631. DOI: 10.1001/archinte.1974.00320160118010

[5] Mohandas N, Gallagher PG. Red cell membrane: Past, present, and future. Blood. 2008;**112**(10):3939-3948. DOI: 10.1182/blood-2008-07-161166

[6] Sesti-Costa R, Costa FF, Conran N. Role of macrophages in sickle cell disease Erythrophagocytosis and erythropoiesis. International Journal of Molecular Sciences. 2023;**24**(7):6333. DOI: 10.3390/ijms24076333

[7] Oldenborg PA, Zheleznyak A, Fang YF, Lagenaur CF, Gresham HD, Lindberg FP. Role of CD47 as a marker of self on red blood cells. Science. 2000;**288**(5473):2051-2054. DOI: 10.1126/science.288.5473.2051

[8] Brousse V, Buffet P, Rees D. The spleen and sickle cell disease: The sick (led) spleen. British Journal of Haematology. 2014;**166**(2):165-176. DOI: 10.1111/bjh.12950

[9] Wandersee NJ, Punzalan RC, Rettig MP, Kennedy MD, Pajewski NM, Sabina RL, et al. Erythrocyte adhesion is modified by alterations in cellular tonicity and volume. British Journal of Haematology. 2005;**131**(3):366-377. DOI: 10.1111/j.1365-2141.2005.05767.x

[10] Platt OS, Falcone JF, Lux SE. Molecular defect in the sickle erythrocyte skeleton. Abnormal spectrin binding to sickle inside-our vesicles. The Journal of Clinical Investigation. 1985;**75**(1):266-271. DOI: 10.1172/JCI111684

[11] Shah R, Taborda C, Chawla S. Acute and chronic hepatobiliary manifestations of sickle cell disease: A review. World Journal of Gastrointestinal Pathophysiology. 2017;**8**(3):108-116. DOI: 10.4291/wjgp.v8.i3.108

[12] Lacaille F, Allali S, de Montalembert M. The liver in sickle cell disease. Journal of Pediatric Gastroenterology and Nutrition. 2021;**72**(1):5-10. DOI: 10.1097/MPG.0000000000002886

[13] Gbotosho OT, Kapetanaki MG, Kato GJ. The worst things in life are free: The role of free Heme in sickle cell disease. Frontiers in Immunology. 2020;**11**:561917. DOI: 10.3389/fimmu.2020.561917

[14] Vallelian F, Buehler PW, Schaer DJ. Hemolysis, free hemoglobin toxicity, and scavenger protein therapeutics. Blood. 2022;**140**(17):1837-1844. DOI: 10.1182/blood.2022015596

[15] Connes P, Alexy T, Detterich J, Romana M, Hardy-Dessources MD, Ballas SK. The role of blood rheology

in sickle cell disease. Blood Reviews. 2016;**30**(2):111-118. DOI: 10.1016/j.blre.2015.08.005

[16] Lang KS, Lang PA, Bauer C, Duranton C, Wieder T, Huber SM, et al. Mechanisms of suicidal erythrocyte death. Cellular Physiology and Biochemistry. 2005;**15**(5):195-202. DOI: 10.1159/000086406

[17] Detterich JA, Liu H, Suriany S, Kato RM, Chalacheva P, Tedla B, et al. Erythrocyte and plasma oxidative stress appears to be compensated in patients with sickle cell disease during a period of relative health, despite the presence of known oxidative agents. Free Radical Biology & Medicine. 2019;**141**:408-415. DOI: 10.1016/j.freeradbiomed.2019.07.004

[18] Antwi-Boasiako C, Dankwah GB, Aryee R, Hayfron-Benjamin C, Donkor ES, Campbell AD. Oxidative profile of patients with sickle cell disease. Medical Sciences (Basel). 2019;**7**(2):17. DOI: 10.3390/medsci7020017

[19] Biswal S, Rizwan H, Pal S, Sabnam S, Parida P, Pal A. Oxidative stress, antioxidant capacity, biomolecule damage, and inflammation symptoms of sickle cell disease in children. Hematology. 2019;**24**(1):1-9. DOI: 10.1080/10245332.2018.1498441

[20] Schacter L, Warth JA, Gordon EM, Prasad A, Klein BL. Altered amount and activity of superoxide dismutase in sickle cell anemia. FASEB Journal. 1988;**2**(3):237-243. DOI: 10.1096/fasebj.2.3.3350236

[21] Morris CR, Suh JH, Hagar W, Larkin S, Bland DA, Steinberg MH, et al. Erythrocyte glutamine depletion, altered redox environment, and pulmonary hypertension in sickle cell disease. Blood. 2008;**111**(1):402-410. DOI: 10.1182/blood-2007-04-081703

[22] Kato GJ, Steinberg MH, Gladwin MT. Intravascular hemolysis and the pathophysiology of sickle cell disease. The Journal of Clinical Investigation. 2017;**127**(3):750-760. DOI: 10.1172/JCI89741

[23] Bozza MT, Jeney V. Pro-inflammatory actions of Heme and other hemoglobin-derived DAMPs. Frontiers in Immunology. 2020;**11**:1323. DOI: 10.3389/fimmu.2020.01323

[24] Reiter CD, Wang X, Tanus-Santos JE, Hogg N, Cannon RO 3rd, Schechter AN, et al. Cell-free hemoglobin limits nitric oxide bioavailability in sickle-cell disease. Nature Medicine. 2002;**8**(12):1383-1389. DOI: 10.1038/nm1202-799

[25] Gladwin MT, Schechter AN, Ognibene FP, Coles WA, Reiter CD, Schenke WH, et al. Divergent nitric oxide bioavailability in men and women with sickle cell disease. Circulation. 2003;**107**(2):271-278. DOI: 10.1161/01.cir.0000044943.12533.a8

[26] Mockesch B, Connes P, Charlot K, Skinner S, Hardy-Dessources MD, Romana M, et al. Association between oxidative stress and vascular reactivity in children with sickle cell anaemia and sickle haemoglobin C disease. British Journal of Haematology. 2017;**178**(3):468-475. DOI: 10.1111/bjh.14693

[27] Hopp MT, Imhof D. Linking labile Heme with thrombosis. Journal of Clinical Medicine. 2021;**10**(3):427. DOI: 10.3390/jcm10030427

[28] Thomsen JH, Etzerodt A, Svendsen P, Moestrup SK. The haptoglobin-CD163-heme oxygenase-1 pathway for hemoglobin scavenging. Oxidative Medicine and Cellular Longevity. 2013;**2013**:523652. DOI: 10.1155/2013/523652

[29] Donegan RK, Moore CM, Hanna DA, Reddi AR. Handling heme: The mechanisms underlying the movement of heme within and between cells. Free Radical Biology & Medicine. 2019;**133**:88-100. DOI: 10.1016/j.freeradbiomed.2018.08.005

[30] Immenschuh S, Vijayan V, Janciauskiene S, Gueler F. Heme as a target for therapeutic interventions. Frontiers in Pharmacology. 2017;**8**:146. DOI: 10.3389/fphar.2017.00146

[31] Ataga KI, Moore CG, Jones S, Olajide O, Strayhorn D, Hinderliter A, et al. Pulmonary hypertension in patients with sickle cell disease: A longitudinal study. British Journal of Haematology. 2006;**134**(1):109-115. DOI: 10.1111/j.1365-2141.2006.06110.x

[32] Minniti CP, Eckman J, Sebastiani P, Steinberg MH, Ballas SK. Leg ulcers in sickle cell disease. American Journal of Hematology. 2010;**85**(10):831-833. DOI: 10.1002/ajh.21838

[33] Wongtong N, Jones S, Deng Y, Cai J, Ataga KI. Monocytosis is associated with hemolysis in sickle cell disease. Hematology. 2015;**20**(10):593-597. DOI: 10.1179/1607845415Y.0000000011

[34] Nickel RS, Osunkwo I, Garrett A, Robertson J, Archer DR, Promislow DE, et al. Immune parameter analysis of children with sickle cell disease on hydroxycarbamide or chronic transfusion therapy. British Journal of Haematology. 2015;**169**(4):574-583. DOI: 10.1111/bjh.13326

[35] Sultana C, Shen Y, Rattan V, Johnson C, Kalra VK. Interaction of sickle erythrocytes with endothelial cells in the presence of endothelial cell conditioned medium induces oxidant stress leading to transendothelial migration of monocytes. Blood. 1998;**92**(10):3924-3935

[36] Belcher JD, Marker PH, Weber JP, Hebbel RP, Vercellotti GM. Activated monocytes in sickle cell disease: Potential role in the activation of vascular endothelium and vaso-occlusion. Blood. 2000;**96**(7):2451-2459. DOI: 10.1182/blood.V96.7.2451

[37] Marcal LE, Dias-da-Motta PM, Rehder J, Mamoni RL, Blotta MH, Whitney CB, et al. Up-regulation of NADPH oxidase components and increased production of interferon-gamma by leukocytes from sickle cell disease patients. American Journal of Hematology. 2008;**83**(1):41-45. DOI: 10.1002/ajh.20991

[38] Ragab SM, Soliman MA. Tissue factor-positive monocytes expression in children with sickle cell disease: Clinical implication and relation to inflammatory and coagulation markers. Blood Coagulation & Fibrinolysis: An International Journal in Haemostasis and Thrombosis. 2016;**27**(8):862-869. DOI: 10.1097/MBC.0000000000000494

[39] Solovey A, Somani A, Belcher JD, Milbauer L, Vincent L, Pawlinski R, et al. A monocyte-TNF-endothelial activation axis in sickle transgenic mice: Therapeutic benefit from TNF blockade. American Journal of Hematology. 2017;**92**(11):1119-1130. DOI: 10.1002/ajh.24856

[40] Inwald DP, Kirkham FJ, Peters MJ, Lane R, Wade A, Evans JP, et al. Platelet and leucocyte activation in childhood sickle cell disease: Association with nocturnal hypoxaemia. British Journal of Haematology. 2000;**111**(2):474-481. DOI: 10.1046/j.1365-2141.2000.02353.x

[41] Wun T, Cordoba M, Rangaswami A, Cheung AW, Paglieroni T. Activated

monocytes and platelet-monocyte aggregates in patients with sickle cell disease. Clinical and Laboratory Haematology. 2002;**24**(2):81-88

[42] Brittain JE, Knoll CM, Ataga KI, Orringer EP, Parise LV. Fibronectin bridges monocytes and reticulocytes via integrin alpha4beta1. British Journal of Haematology. 2008;**141**(6):872-881. DOI: 10.1111/j.1365-2141.2008.07056.x

[43] Liu Y, Jing F, Yi W, Mendelson A, Shi P, Walsh R, et al. HO-1(hi) patrolling monocytes protect against vaso-occlusion in sickle cell disease. Blood. 2018;**131**(14):1600-1610. DOI: 10.1182/blood-2017-12-819870

[44] Vinchi F, Costa da Silva M, Ingoglia G, Petrillo S, Brinkman N, Zuercher A, et al. Hemopexin therapy reverts heme-induced proinflammatory phenotypic switching of macrophages in a mouse model of sickle cell disease. Blood. 2016;**127**(4):473-486. DOI: 10.1182/blood-2015-08-663245

[45] Dutra FF, Alves LS, Rodrigues D, Fernandez PL, de Oliveira RB, Golenbock DT, et al. Hemolysis-induced lethality involves inflammasome activation by heme. Proceedings of the National Academy of Sciences of the United States of America. 2014;**111**(39):E4110-E4118. DOI: 10.1073/pnas.1405023111

[46] Anyaegbu CC, Okpala IE, Akren'Ova YA, Salimonu LS. Peripheral blood neutrophil count and candidacidal activity correlate with the clinical severity of sickle cell anaemia (SCA). European Journal of Haematology. 1998;**60**(4):267-268

[47] Almeida CB, Scheiermann C, Jang JE, Prophete C, Costa FF, Conran N, et al. Hydroxyurea and a cGMP-amplifying agent have immediate benefits on acute vaso-occlusive events in sickle cell disease mice. Blood. 2012;**120**(14):2879-2888. DOI: 10.1182/blood-2012-02-409524

[48] Benkerrou M, Delarche C, Brahimi L, Fay M, Vilmer E, Elion J, et al. Hydroxyurea corrects the dysregulated L-selectin expression and increased H(2)O(2) production of polymorphonuclear neutrophils from patients with sickle cell anemia. Blood. 2002;**99**(7):2297-2303

[49] Koehl B, Nivoit P, El Nemer W, Lenoir O, Hermand P, Pereira C, et al. The endothelin B receptor plays a crucial role in the adhesion of neutrophils to the endothelium in sickle cell disease. Haematologica. 2017;**102**(7):1161-1172. DOI: 10.3324/haematol.2016.156869

[50] Turhan A, Weiss LA, Mohandas N, Coller BS, Frenette PS. Primary role for adherent leukocytes in sickle cell vascular occlusion: A new paradigm. Proceedings of the National Academy of Sciences of the United States of America. 2002;**99**(5):3047-3051. DOI: 10.1073/pnas.052522799

[51] Zhang D, Xu C, Manwani D, Frenette PS. Neutrophils, platelets, and inflammatory pathways at the nexus of sickle cell disease pathophysiology. Blood. 2016;**127**(7):801-809. DOI: 10.1182/blood-2015-09-618538

[52] Ataga KI, Kutlar A, Kanter J, Liles D, Cancado R, Friedrisch J, et al. Crizanlizumab for the prevention of pain crises in sickle cell disease. The New England Journal of Medicine. 2017;**376**(5):429-439. DOI: 10.1056/NEJMoa1611770

[53] Telen MJ, Wun T, McCavit TL, De Castro LM, Krishnamurti L, Lanzkron S, et al. Randomized phase 2 study of GMI-1070 in SCD: Reduction in time to resolution of vaso-occlusive events

and decreased opioid use. Blood. 2015;**125**(17):2656-2664. DOI: 10.1182/blood-2014-06-583351

[54] Zhang D, Chen G, Manwani D, Mortha A, Xu C, Faith JJ, et al. Neutrophil ageing is regulated by the microbiome. Nature. 2015;**525**(7570):528-532. DOI: 10.1038/nature15367

[55] Ghosh S, Adisa OA, Chappa P, Tan F, Jackson KA, Archer DR, et al. Extracellular hemin crisis triggers acute chest syndrome in sickle mice. The Journal of Clinical Investigation. 2013;**123**(11):4809-4820. DOI: 10.1172/JCI64578

[56] Afrin LB. Mast cell activation syndrome as a significant comorbidity in sickle cell disease. The American Journal of the Medical Sciences. 2014;**348**(6):460-464. DOI: 10.1097/MAJ.0000000000000325

[57] Allali S, Lionnet F, Mattioni S, Callebert J, Stankovic Stojanovic K, Bachmeyer C, et al. Plasma histamine elevation in a large cohort of sickle cell disease patients. British Journal of Haematology. 2019;**186**(1):125-129. DOI: 10.1111/bjh.15900

[58] Brandow AM, Wandersee NJ, Dasgupta M, Hoffmann RG, Hillery CA, Stucky CL, et al. Substance P is increased in patients with sickle cell disease and associated with haemolysis and hydroxycarbamide use. British Journal of Haematology. 2016;**175**(2):237-245. DOI: 10.1111/bjh.14300

[59] Vincent L, Vang D, Nguyen J, Gupta M, Luk K, Ericson ME, et al. Mast cell activation contributes to sickle cell pathobiology and pain in mice. Blood. 2013;**122**(11):1853-1862. DOI: 10.1182/blood-2013-04-498105

[60] Federti E, Matte A, Recchiuti A, Garello F, Ghigo A, El Nemer W, et al. In humanized sickle cell mice, Imatinib protects against sickle cell-related injury. Hema. 2023;**7**(3):e848. DOI: 10.1097/HS9.0000000000000848

[61] Karimi M, Bahadoram M, Mafakher L, Rastegar M. Impact of Imatinib on reducing the painful crisis in patients with sickle cell disease. Hematology, Transfusion and Cell Therapy. 2023. pp. 1-6. DOI: 10.1016/j.htct.2023.06.007

[62] Mold C, Tamerius JD, Phillips G Jr. Complement activation during painful crisis in sickle cell anemia. Clinical Immunology and Immunopathology. 1995;**76**(3 Pt 1):314-320. DOI: 10.1006/clin.1995.1131

[63] Wang RH, Phillips G Jr, Medof ME, Mold C. Activation of the alternative complement pathway by exposure of phosphatidylethanolamine and phosphatidylserine on erythrocytes from sickle cell disease patients. The Journal of Clinical Investigation. 1993;**92**(3):1326-1335. DOI: 10.1172/JCI116706

[64] Test ST, Woolworth VS. Defective regulation of complement by the sickle erythrocyte: Evidence for a defect in control of membrane attack complex formation. Blood. 1994;**83**(3):842-852

[65] Roumenina LT, Chadebech P, Bodivit G, Vieira-Martins P, Grunenwald A, Boudhabhay I, et al. Complement activation in sickle cell disease: Dependence on cell density, hemolysis and modulation by hydroxyurea therapy. American Journal of Hematology. 2020;**95**(5):456-464. DOI: 10.1002/ajh.25742

[66] Merle NS, Grunenwald A, Rajaratnam H, Gnemmi V, Frimat M, Figueres ML, et al. Intravascular hemolysis activates complement via cell-free heme and

heme-loaded microvesicles. JCI Insight. 2018;**3**(12):e96910. DOI: 10.1172/jci.insight.96910

[67] Lombardi E, Matte A, Risitano AM, Ricklin D, Lambris JD, De Zanet D, et al. Factor H interferes with the adhesion of sickle red cells to vascular endothelium: A novel disease-modulating molecule. Haematologica. 2019;**104**(5):919-928. DOI: 10.3324/haematol.2018.198622

[68] Meuleman MS, Roumenina LT, Grunenwald A. Complement involvement in sickle cell disease. Presse Médicale. 2023;**52**(4):104205. DOI: 10.1016/j.lpm.2023.104205

[69] Belcher JD, Chen C, Nguyen J, Milbauer L, Abdulla F, Alayash AI, et al. Heme triggers TLR4 signaling leading to endothelial cell activation and vaso-occlusion in murine sickle cell disease. Blood. 2014;**123**(3):377-390. DOI: 10.1182/blood-2013-04-495887

[70] Erdei J, Toth A, Balogh E, Nyakundi BB, Banyai E, Ryffel B, et al. Induction of NLRP3 Inflammasome activation by Heme in human endothelial cells. Oxidative Medicine and Cellular Longevity. 2018;**2018**:4310816. DOI: 10.1155/2018/4310816

[71] Belcher JD, Zhang P, Nguyen J, Kiser ZM, Nath KA, Hu J, et al. Identification of a Heme activation site on the MD-2/TLR4 complex. Frontiers in Immunology. 2020;**11**:1370. DOI: 10.3389/fimmu.2020.01370

[72] Zhang P, Nguyen J, Abdulla F, Nelson AT, Beckman JD, Vercellotti GM, et al. Soluble MD-2 and Heme in sickle cell disease plasma promote pro-inflammatory signaling in endothelial cells. Frontiers in Immunology. 2021;**12**:632709. DOI: 10.3389/fimmu.2021.632709

[73] Allali S, Rignault-Bricard R, de Montalembert M, Taylor M, Bouceba T, Hermine O, et al. HbS promotes TLR4-mediated monocyte activation and proinflammatory cytokine production in sickle cell disease. Blood. 2022;**140**(18):1972-1982. DOI: 10.1182/blood.2021014894

[74] Liu Y, Pal M, Bao W, Shi PA, Lobo CA, An X, et al. Type I interferon is induced by hemolysis and drives antibody-mediated erythrophagocytosis in sickle cell disease. Blood. 2021;**138**(13):1162-1171. DOI: 10.1182/blood.2021011629

[75] Gladwin MT, Vichinsky E. Pulmonary complications of sickle cell disease. The New England Journal of Medicine. 2008;**359**(21):2254-2265. DOI: 10.1056/NEJMra0804411

[76] Vichinsky EP, Styles LA, Colangelo LH, Wright EC, Castro O, Nickerson B. Acute chest syndrome in sickle cell disease: Clinical presentation and course. Cooperative study of sickle cell disease. Blood. 1997;**89**(5):1787-1792. DOI: DOI

[77] Hunter CA, Jones SA. IL-6 as a keystone cytokine in health and disease. Nature Immunology. 2015;**16**(5):448-457. DOI: 10.1038/ni.3153

[78] Allali S, de Montalembert M, Rignault-Bricard R, Taylor M, Brice J, Brousse V, et al. IL-6 levels are dramatically high in the sputum from children with sickle cell disease during acute chest syndrome. Blood Advances. 2020;**4**(24):6130-6134. DOI: 10.1182/bloodadvances.2020003519

[79] Allali S, Elie J, Mayrand L, de Montalembert M, Taylor M, Brice J, et al. Sputum IL-6 level as a potential predictor of acute chest syndrome during vaso-occlusive crisis in children

with sickle cell disease: Exploratory prospective prognostic accuracy study. American Journal of Hematology. 2023;**98**(7):E175-E178. DOI: 10.1002/ajh.26939

[80] Allali S, Chhun S, de Montalembert M, Heilbronner C, Taylor M, Brice J, et al. Tocilizumab for severe acute chest syndrome in a child with sickle cell disease and dramatically high interleukin-6 values in endotracheal and pleural fluids. American Journal of Hematology. 2022;**97**(3):E81-E83. DOI: 10.1002/ajh.26433

Chapter 2

Emerging Trends in Sickle Cell Disease and CRISPR/Caspases

Grace K. Ababio

Abstract

In this review chapter, sickle cell disease (SCD) overview, its diagnostic procedures and markers to date as well as the proposed model or pathways by which SCD oxidative stress activates caspases leading to a shrunken sickle cell are presented. Of the various approaches used to mitigate SCD effects, it is anticipated that the Clustered Regularly Interspaced Short Palindromic Repeats (CRISPR)/Caspases could possibly edit the sixth position alteration on the β-globin gene on chromosome 11. Even though CRISPR/Caspases hold promise in sickle cell disease in the near future, it is also possible for it to create genomic chaos. Here, several schools of thought are presented as well.

Keywords: sickle cell disease, diagnostics, haplotypes, oxidative stress, inflammatory marker, CRISPR, caspases

1. Introduction

SCD is the commonest hemoglobinopathy [1] affecting millions of people worldwide and this remains a public health concern. The disease evolved through four periods: the tribal medicine period in Africa [2], clinical recognition by Western medicine, an era of biochemical/molecular characterization [3, 4] with Venon Mason and Linus Pauling initiative [5, 6], and now an era of molecular therapy [7].

Even though SCD can cause extravascular and intravascular hemolysis [8, 9], it is normally characterized by normocytic intrinsic hemolytic anemia [10] brought on by defective hemoglobin and erythrocytes. Defective hemoglobin is due to a deficient zinc [11, 12] that does not favor hemoglobin binding to increase oxygen affinity. The defect is actually an amino acid alteration at the sixth position of the beta (β)-globin subunit on chromosome 11 [13]. This paves the way for an autosomal recessive inheritance [14].

Aside from this, SCD is a multifactorial disease-causing organ damage from acute events and or subacute events with a progression of chronic SCD. SCD displays phenotypic variability with severer and or life-threatening consequences with the hallmark being vaso-occlusive crisis (VOC) [15].

Several variants of SCD types exist with diverse disease presentations. For instance, HbAS is asymptomatic, as HbSC and HbCC have milder presentation while HbSS remains the severe form. In HbSS, elevated altitude, decreased oxygen, and or acidosis precipitate the sickling status [16]. HbF protects newborns with the defect from zero to 6 months [17, 18]. Individuals with the trait (heterozygotes) appear resistant to malaria.

A myriad of SCD complications do exist [19], namely, autosplenectomy, aplastic crisis, splenic infarction or sequestration crisis, dactylitis, acute chest syndrome, hematuria, renal papillary necrosis, priapism, and bacterial infection, e.g., *Salmonella spp.*

2. Diagnostic methods

Microscopy, full blood count, hemoglobin electrophoresis, high-performance liquid chromatography (HPLC) [20], and skull X-rays are popular diagnostic methods used in detecting SCD status. From full blood count, low hemoglobin levels, high white blood cell count, high reticulocyte count, increased hematocrit, and possible platelet count increase are observed. On skull x-ray, "Crew cut" shape is seen due to bone marrow expansion from elevated erythropoiesis. On microscopic slides, sickle cells appear crescent-shaped. Even though cellulose acetate electrophoresis (**Figure 1**)

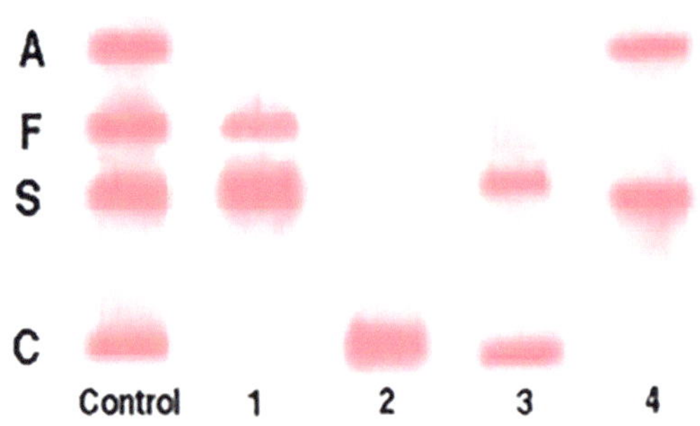

Figure 1.
Cellulose acetate electrophoresis from authors lab.

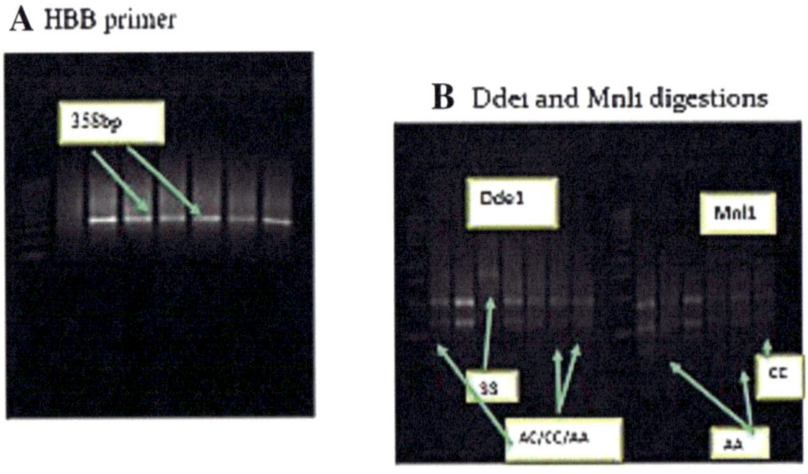

Figure 2.
Electrophoretogram from author's lab [23]. Gel A shows 358 bp band size of the β-globin gene and gel B shows RFLP sizes of Dde1 and Mnl1 endonucleases. A 100 bp DNA ladder was used.

remains the highly utilized approach, possible molecular sieving effects seem to be a limiting factor. The cellulose acetate membrane is marked and made wet with an alkaline buffer prior to the start of the experiment. Saline (0.85%) washed red blood cells are placed at vantage points on the membrane; voltage and time are then set for the electrophoretic run. The migration of hemoglobin is determined by comparison to a reference hemoglobinopathy.

Starch–polyacrylamide gel electrophoresis was a chanced upon approach that provided a good resolution in author's lab in a bid to investigate glyoxalase phenotypes in diabetes [21], however, electro-osmotic effect and variation in starch pore size from batch to batch was found to be the biggest challenge. In this chanced approach, hemolyzed red blood cells were run on a discontinuous 7.5% polyacrylamide and 0.3% hydrolyzed starch with pH being 8.8 and a non-starch stacking gel with pH being 6.8. Tris-glycine, pH 8.9 was the electrophoretic buffer and the electrophoresis was performed for 2 hrs, 100 V, 55 mA at room temperature.

Even though starch–polyacrylamide gel electrophoresis (PAGE) was not extensively explored in SCD, it gives very good resolution with the exception of it being expensive, laborious and time-consuming.

Polymerase chain reaction [22], restriction fragment polymorphisms (RFLP, **Figure 2**) [23] and single nucleotide polymorphisms [24, 25] were also explored, but these approaches were very expensive, laborious and time consuming as well.

For polymerase chain reaction, a 1 μl DNA, 2 μM of each primer set, 0.2 mM of each dNTP, 1 unit of DNA Hotstart polymerase and a buffer containing 2.5 mM $MgCl_2$ making a total of 20 μl was set for PCR reaction mix. Thermal cycling conditions included a 94°C for 15 minutes, 45 cycles involving 94°C for 30 sec, followed by 62°C for 30 sec and then 72°C for 60 sec with a final lengthening at 72°C for 10 minutes. PCR products were then run on 1.5% agarose gel electrophoresis and visualized with the imager. The forward 5′-AGGAGCAGGGAGGGCAGGA-3′ and reverse primer 5′-CCAAGGGTAGACCACCAGC-3′ were able to give 358 bp PCR product which paved the way for Mnl1 and Dde I restriction enzymes to discriminate between the hemoglobin genotypes in RFLP. All RFLPs followed the manufacturer's protocol and were resolved on 3% agarose gels.

3. Markers of SCD till date

Restriction endonucleases which were consistent with literature paved way for the determination of β-globin gene cluster of haplotypes in the author's lab (article has reached publication stage). These haplotypes were Senegal, Benin, Bantu, Cameroon, and Arab-Indian [26]. This came to light when certain haplotypes were linked to SCD clinical outcomes [27]. However, phenotypic variation seems to be a limiting factor among individuals with common haplotype causing the previous notion to be seemingly unreliable despite the high hopes of presumptive predictors of disease severity for optimal treatment.

Revolutionized methods also, only depicted historical value and or logistic constraints. Identified biochemical and clinical biomarkers are also not routinely incorporated in SCD care algorithms. Notwithstanding, extensive work on inflammatory markers [28–30] gained strides in SCD. Yet, there seems to be no reliable marker for SCD pain except vaso occlusive crisis, its hallmark.

4. The paradigm shift

Of the varying approaches used in alleviating painful SCD outcomes, hydroxyurea [31], folate analogs [32], zinc supplements [33], transfusion and gene therapy [34] remain the widely utilized methods. SCD patients are zinc deficient, thus zinc supplementation remains an important approach in the treatment. Folate analogs on the other hand, inhibit dihydrofolate reductase in DNA synthesis. Hydroxyurea inhibits thymidylate synthase and promotes the release of tumor necrosis factor (TNF alpha). TNF alpha, a pro-inflammatory cytokine is involved in the ligand-receptor interactions of the extrinsic mitochondrial apoptotic pathway in SCD.

Following the intrinsic mitochondrial apoptotic pathway closely, it is anticipated and proposed in this write-up that oxidative stress can cause cytochrome C to be released from the mitochondria and cytochrome C will in turn activate the caspases which can duly alter cell shape (**Figure 3**).

However, a new paradigm shift which is currently being considered is CRISPR/caspases in gene therapy.

5. CRISPR/caspases and SCD

CRISPR, a gene editing tool that made its discoverers, Doudna and Charpentier [35], received the Nobel prize, and is obtained from bacteria. It contains a guide RNA (gRNA) [36] and an endonuclease (caspase e.g., Cas9), which makes strand breaks at target sites. Thus, gene knock-outs or knock-ins could be created on chromosome 11,

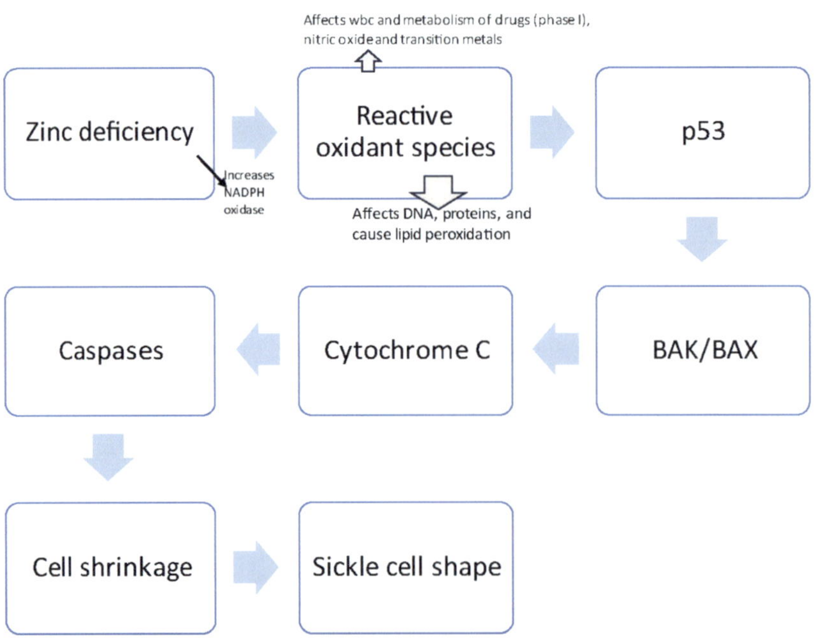

Figure 3.
The proposed intrinsic mitochondrial apoptotic model by which SCD oxidative stress activate caspases leading to an altered cell shape. All arrows indicate stimulation or activation. Activated p53 induces cell cycle arrest and promote DNA repair and/or apoptosis. BAK/BAX regulate apoptotic caspase system. Cytochrome C is an important candidate in the life-supporting function of ATP synthesis (the energy currency).

Manifestation	Objective	Target	Sponsor	Trial ID	Reference
Sickle cell disease (SCD)	Increase fetal hemoglobin	BCL11A and Cas9 reinforcement	Vertex Pharm. and CRISPR therapeutics	NCT03745287	[37]
transfusion-dependent β-thalassemia (TDT)	Increase HbF	Improving Cas9 and BCL11A	CRISPR therapy and Vertex Pharmaceuticals	NCT03655678	[37]
SCD	Elevate HbF	ZFN and BCL11A enhancer	Sangamo Therapeutics and Sanofi	NCT03653247	[38–40]
TDT	Improve HbF levels	BCL11A and ZFN reinforcer	Sanofi and Sangamo Therapeutics	NCT03432364	[38–40]

Other collaborators like Intellia Therapeutics, Novartis, Graphite Bio, UCSF Benioffs, UCLA and IGI have ongoing trials with the same objectives but are yet to receive the clinical trial ID.

Table 1.
CRISPR SCD clinical trials.

the β-globin gene, ensuring desirable outcomes in SCD. However, editing the SCD gene might require a dedicated and reliable facility to confine subjects for the necessary procedure as well as financial obligations.

Sponsorships and or collaborators from pharmaceuticals like Sanofi, Vertex, Sangamo, and CRISPR therapeutics have ongoing clinical trials with a recognizable ID; while collaborators like Intellia Therapeutics, Graphite Bio, Novartis, UCSF Benioffs, IGI, and UCLA are yet to obtain IDs for their ongoing trials (**Table 1**), [37–40]. All these SCD clinical trials do have the same goal and this is to increase fetal hemoglobin levels (**Table 1**), [37–40]. The successful SCD clinical trials that utilized few subjects ranging from four to eight individuals seem not to have extensively involved off – target (the clinic – scale approach) and indels. Indels could be obtained from next-generation sequencing. Thus, it is therefore unsure of the possible clonal formation from indels.

Also, despite the fact that desirable events like homology-directed repair and non-homologous end joining remain the main goals of CRISPR/caspases, it is thus, possible to generate undesirable or unwanted events. Concerns on CRISPR/Cas9 had been on off-target activity [41]. However, several mechanisms to detect or predict risk as well as to reduce risk [42] have been proposed.

Yet still, according to Amendola et al. it is possible to generate micronuclei (for instance, GTG banding and fluorescence *in situ* hybridization could pick up micronuclei) [43–45] and chromosomal bridges since one cannot quantify cell cycle in hematopoietic stem cell at the time of transplantation. Also, if rearrangements of chromosomes (such as 1- to 50-kb inversions/deletions, chromosome truncations, translocations, and combinations of these rearrangements) occur in progenitor cells, it is possible for unwanted event to occur.

6. Conclusion

In this write-up, it was indicated that, even though CRISPR/Cas9 holds the promise of modeling SCD for effective gene therapy, the unanticipated chaos for clinical applications should not be ignored. Much work is needed in this regard as we strive toward excellence in SCD treatments.

Author details

Grace K. Ababio
Medical Biochemistry, University of Ghana Medical School, Korle-Bu, Accra, Ghana

*Address all correspondence to: gkababio@ug.edu.gh

References

[1] Park KW. Sickle cell disease and other hemoglobinopathies. International Anesthesiology Clinics. 2004;**42**(3):77-93

[2] Onwubalili J. Sickle-cell anaemia: An explanation for the ancient myth of reincarnation in Nigeria. The Lancet. 1983;**322**(8348):503-505

[3] Abboud MR, Musallam KM. Sickle cell disease at the dawn of the molecular era. Hemoglobin. 2009;**33**(sup1):S93-S106

[4] Steinberg MH. Sickle cell anemia, the first molecular disease: Overview of molecular etiology, pathophysiology, and therapeutic approaches. The Scientific World Journal. 2008;**8**:1295-1324

[5] Pauling L, Itano HA, Singer SJ, Wells IC. Sickle cell anemia, a molecular disease. Science. 1949;**110**:543-548

[6] Ingram V. A specific chemical difference between the globins of normal human and sickle-cell anaemia haemoglobin. Nature. 1956;**178**:79

[7] Hoban MD, Orkin SH, Bauer DE. Genetic treatment of a molecular disorder: Gene therapy approaches to sickle cell disease. Blood, The Journal of the American Society of Hematology. 2016;**127**(7):839-848

[8] Kato GJ, Gladwin MT. Mechanisms and clinical complications of hemolysis in sickle cell disease and thalassemia. Disorders of Hemoglobin: Genetics, Pathophysiology, and Clinical Management. 2009;**2**:201-224

[9] Kato GJ, Steinberg MH, Gladwin MT. Intravascular hemolysis and the pathophysiology of sickle cell disease. The Journal of Clinical Investigation. 2017;**127**(3):750-760

[10] Kavanagh PL, Fasipe TA, Wun T. Sickle cell disease: a review. JAMA. 2022;**328**(1):57-68

[11] Prasad AS. Zinc deficiency in patients with sickle cell disease. The American Journal of Clinical Nutrition. 2002;**75**(2):181-182

[12] Prasad AS, Schoomaker EB, Ortega J, Brewer GJ, Oberleas D, Oelshlegel FJ Jr. Zinc deficiency in sickle cell disease. Clinical Chemistry. 1975;**21**(4):582-587

[13] Adekile A. The genetic and clinical significance of fetal hemoglobin expression in sickle cell disease. Medical Principles and Practice. 2021;**30**(3):201-211

[14] Ogedegbe HO. Sickle cell disease: An overview. Laboratory Medicine. 2002;**33**(7):515-543

[15] Ballas SK. Pathophysiology and principles of management of the many faces of the acute vaso-occlusive crisis in patients with sickle cell disease. European Journal of Haematology. 2015;**95**(2):113-123

[16] Tewari S, Brousse V, Piel FB, Menzel S, Rees DC. Environmental determinants of severity in sickle cell disease. Haematologica. 2015;**100**(9):1108

[17] Conran N. High foetal haemoglobin in sickle cell disease: Not so protective? eBioMedicine. 2015;**2**(2):102-103

[18] Steinberg MH. Fetal hemoglobin in sickle hemoglobinopathies: High HbF genotypes and phenotypes. Journal of Clinical Medicine. 2020;**9**(11):3782

[19] Ogu UO, Billett HH. Comorbidities in sickle cell disease: Adult providers

needed! The Indian Journal of Medical Research. 2018;**147**(6):527

[20] Ray GK, Jena RK. Spectrum of hemoglobinopathies: A new revelation in a tertiary care hospital of Odisha. Indian Journal of Hematology and Blood Transfusion. 2019;**35**:513-517

[21] Amanquah S, Aleksenko L, Ababio G, Ankrah NA, Quaye IK. Red cell glyoxalase 1 polymorphism in Ghanaians: A report of new variants. International Journal of Medical and Applied Sciences. 2014;**3**(3):123-128

[22] Singh PJ, Shrivastava AC, Shrikhande AV. Prenatal diagnosis of sickle cell disease by the technique of PCR. Indian Journal of Hematology and Blood Transfusion. 2015;**31**:233-241

[23] Tripathi GR. A simplified and cheapest method for the diagnosis of sickle cell using whole blood PCR and RFLP in Nepal. Tribhuvan University Journal. 2016;**30**(2):57-64

[24] Fertrin KY, Costa FF. Genomic polymorphisms in sickle cell disease: Implications for clinical diversity and treatment. Expert Review of Hematology. 2010;**3**(4):443-458

[25] Ababio GK, Ekem I, Acquaye J, Oppong SY, Amoah AGB, Brandful J, et al. Detection of transversions and transitions in HBG2 cis-elements associated with sickle cell allele in Ghanaians. Biochemical Genetics. 2023:1-9. DOI: 10.1007/s10528-023-10438-1. PMID: 37395849

[26] Al-Ali AK, Alsulaiman A, Alzahrani AJ, Obeid OT, Vatte CB, Cyrus C, et al. Prevalence and diversity of haplotypes of sickle cell disease in the Eastern Province of Saudi Arabia. Hemoglobin. 2020;**44**(2):78-81

[27] Rusanova I, Escames G, Cossio G, De Borace RG, Moreno B, Chahboune M, et al. Oxidative stress status, clinical outcome, and β-globin gene cluster haplotypes in pediatric patients with sickle cell disease. European Journal of Haematology. 2010;**85**(6):529-537

[28] Rees DC, Gibson JS. Biomarkers in sickle cell disease. British Journal of Haematology. 2012;**156**(4):433-445

[29] Damanhouri GA, Jarullah J, Marouf S, Hindawi SI, Mushtaq G, Kamal MA. Clinical biomarkers in sickle cell disease. Saudi Journal of Biological Sciences. 2015;**22**(1):24-31

[30] Conran N, Belcher JD. Inflammation in sickle cell disease. Clinical Hemorheology and Microcirculation. 2018;**68**(2-3):263-299

[31] Nevitt SJ, Jones AP, Howard J. Hydroxyurea (hydroxycarbamide) for sickle cell disease. Cochrane Database of Systematic Reviews. 2017;**4**:CD002202

[32] Ballas SK. Sickle cell disease: Current clinical management. In: Seminars in Hematology. Vol. 38, No. 4. Philadelphia, PA, USA: WB Saunders; 2001. pp. 307-314

[33] Bao B, Prasad AS, Beck FW, Snell D, Suneja A, Sarkar FH, et al. Zinc supplementation decreases oxidative stress, incidence of infection, and generation of inflammatory cytokines in sickle cell disease patients. Translational Research. 2008;**152**(2):67-80

[34] Ribeil JA, Hacein-Bey-Abina S, Payen E, Magnani A, Semeraro M, Magrin E, et al. Gene therapy in a patient with sickle cell disease. New England Journal of Medicine. 2017;**376**(9):848-855

[35] Jinek M, Chylinski K, Fonfara I, et al. A programmable dual-RNA-guided

DNA endonuclease in adaptive bacterial immunity. Science. 2012;**337**:816-821. DOI: 10.1126/science.1225829

[36] Hu C, van Beljouw SP, Nam KH, Schuler G, Ding F, Cui Y, et al. Craspase is a CRISPR RNA-guided, RNA-activated protease. Science. 2022;**377**(6612):1278-1285

[37] Canver MC, Smith EC, Sher F, Pinello L, Sanjana NE, Shalem O, et al. BCL11A enhancer dissection by Cas9-mediated in situ saturating mutagenesis. Nature. 2015;**527**(7577):192-197

[38] Vierstra J, Reik A, Chang KH, Stehling-Sun S, Zhou Y, Hinkley SJ, et al. Functional footprinting of regulatory DNA. Nature Methods. 2015;**12**(10):927-930

[39] Chang KH, Smith SE, Sullivan T, Chen K, Zhou Q, West JA, et al. Long-term engraftment and fetal globin induction upon BCL11A gene editing in bone-marrow-derived CD34+ hematopoietic stem and progenitor cells. Molecular Therapy-Methods & Clinical Development. 2017;**4**:137-148

[40] Psatha N, Reik A, Phelps S, Zhou Y, Dalas D, Yannaki E, et al. Disruption of the BCL11A erythroid enhancer reactivates fetal hemoglobin in erythroid cells of patients with β-thalassemia major. Molecular Therapy-Methods & Clinical Development. 2018;**10**:313-326

[41] Fu Y, Foden JA, Khayter C, et al. High-frequency off-target mutagenesis induced by CRISPR-Cas nucleases in human cells. Nature Biotechnology. 2013;**31**:822-826. DOI: 10.1038/nbt.2623

[42] Tsai SQ, Joung JK. Defining and improving the genome wide specificities of CRISPR-Cas9 nucleases. Nature Reviews. Genetics. 2016;**17**:300-312. DOI: 10.1038/nrg.2016.28

[43] Boutin J, Cappellen D, Rosier J, et al. ON-target adverse events of CRISPR-Cas9 nuclease: More chaotic than expected. CRISPR Journal. 2022;**5**:19-30. DOI: 10.1089/crispr.2021.0120

[44] Teboul L, Herault Y, Wells S, et al. Variability in genome editing outcomes: Challenges for research reproducibility and clinical safety. Molecular Therapy. 2020;**28**:1422-1431. DOI: 10.1016/j.ymthe.2020.03.015

[45] Amendola M, Brusson M, Miccio A. CRISPRthripsis: The risk of CRISPR/Cas9-induced chromothripsis in gene therapy. Stem Cells Translational Medicine. 2022;**11**(10):1003-1009

Chapter 3

Cardiopulmonary Complications of Sickle Cell Disease in Children

Maria Teresa Santiago, Lance Feld, Arushi Dhar, La Nyka Christian-Weekes, Abena Appiah-Kubi, Elizabeth Mitchell, Banu Aygun and Elizabeth K. Fiorino

Abstract

Sickle cell disease (SCD) is an autosomal recessive hemoglobinopathy leading to hemolysis, increased endothelial adhesion, inflammation, and vasculopathy. While most children with SCD have normal pulmonary function, lung capacity and expiratory flows are lower compared to age- and racially matched controls. Airway obstruction dominates in children, with restrictive ventilatory defects becoming more prevalent in adolescents and young adults. Decreased pulmonary function, physician-diagnosed asthma, airway hyperresponsiveness, wheezing, and sleep-disordered breathing are associated with more frequent episodes of acute chest syndrome and vaso-occlusive crisis. Chronic lung disease, thromboembolism, hypoxemia, and sleep-disordered breathing are associated with the development of pulmonary hypertension and ventricular dysfunction which carry significant morbidity and mortality risk in adults. Most treatments for cardiopulmonary complications of SCD are based on guidelines developed for the general population. Although most guidelines do not recommend routine screening of asymptomatic children, patients with cardiopulmonary symptoms should be monitored and treated by subspecialists in a multidisciplinary setting. Disease modifying treatments such as hydroxyurea are attenuating some of the cardiopulmonary complications in SCD. More studies need to be done to assess the effects of newer disease modifying treatments targeting hemolysis and decreasing endothelial adhesion.

Keywords: child, complications, treatment, acute chest syndrome, pulmonary function, asthma, sleep-disordered breathing, ventricular dysfunction, pulmonary hypertension

1. Introduction

Sickle cell disease (SCD) is a hemoglobinopathy resulting from mutations in the β-globin gene and is inherited in an autosomal recessive pattern [1]. Public health measures in developed countries have helped improve infant morbidity and mortality; however, the long-term complications from this condition represent a global health burden [2]. The point mutation in SCD is a substitution of valine for glutamic acid at the sixth position of the β-globin gene resulting in "sickled" hemoglobin that is less soluble than normal adult or fetal hemoglobin (HbF). With deoxygenation, hemoglobin S becomes polymerized resulting in decreased erythrocyte flexibility forming the characteristic "sickled" shape. These changes alter cellular function, enhance endothelial adhesion molecule expression, impair microvascular flow, and promote hemolysis and vaso-occlusion leading to anemia, hemolysis, vasculopathy, and chronic inflammation [1]. Cardiopulmonary involvement is a major cause of morbidity and mortality in adults. There is growing evidence suggesting earlier onset of pulmonary function abnormalities, and predisposition to disorders, such as asthma, thromboembolism, sleep-disordered breathing (SDB), ventricular dysfunction, and pulmonary hypertension, in children with SCD [3–5]. It is the aim of this narrative review to summarize current literature describing cardiopulmonary complications of SCD in children and evolving treatments that may improve outcomes.

2. Acute chest syndrome

Acute chest syndrome (ACS) is a known complication of SCD with high morbidity and mortality. Newer data suggest that repeated episodes of ACS may be associated with decreased lung function longitudinally in children, and increased inflammation [6]. Key factors in the pathogenesis of ACS include pulmonary infection, pulmonary infarction, and fat embolism. Identification of exact infectious etiology in children varies and can be identified in over two-thirds of cases, with viruses predominating [7]. Of note, since the initiation of pneumococcal vaccination with PCV-13 (13-valent pneumococcal conjugate vaccine), one cohort in France demonstrated a 41.8% decrease in ACS over time [8]. Diagnosis is clinical, and criteria are the following: new infiltrate on chest X-ray, hypoxemia, and respiratory signs/symptoms [1]. Treatment involves supplemental oxygen, empiric antibiotics to cover *Mycoplasma pneumoniae* and encapsulated organisms, chest physiotherapy and incentive spirometry, pain control, and, when indicated, transfusion and ventilatory support [9].

3. Pulmonary function abnormalities

Pulmonary function abnormalities have been demonstrated in infants and children with SCD. Koumbourlis et al. [10] found evidence of lower airway obstruction and hyperinflation in 20 infants (aged 3–30 months) with SCD, particularly those with homozygous sickle cell disease (HbSS). Functional Residual Capacity (FRC) was elevated, maximum expiratory flow rates at FRC and time to reach peak expiratory flow were decreased. A cross-sectional study of 22 infants, 6–18 months of age, showed evidence of obstruction, independent of acute chest syndrome (ACS) or vaso-occlusive events (VOE). The investigators found normal lung function in 77% of infants with SCD but lower Forced Vital Capacity (FVC), lower forced expiratory flow at 0.5 seconds (FEF0.5), and forced expiratory flow at 25 to 75% of FVC (FEF25–75) compared with controls [11].

Despite the frequency of respiratory complaints in patients with SCD, longitudinal studies spanning progression of pulmonary function abnormalities from childhood to adulthood are limited. Cross-sectional studies reveal that 70–80% of school-aged children with SCD have normal lung function but values are reduced compared to age-, gender-, and race-matched healthy controls. Although international guidelines recommend the use of lower-limit-of-normal (LLN) criteria (which can vary by age, height, and gender) to define abnormal lung function, several studies on children with SCD use cutoffs (such as a forced expiratory volume in 1 second (FEV1)/FVC < 0.70 or % predicted values below 80%) to distinguish normal versus abnormal [5]. Airway obstruction is the most common abnormality found in children (16–34%). Restrictive defects, which are usually found in adults with SCD, have been described less frequently in children (2–11%) [4, 5, 12–15]. It is not known if lung deficits in SCD are secondary to underlying airway inflammation or a result of pulmonary injury following ACS or allergic disease [6]. Data from the Sleep and Asthma Cohort (SAC) showed that lung function patterns (obstruction, restriction, and nonspecific ventilatory defects) were not associated with future pain or ACS episodes over a 4-year follow-up period [15]. In a meta-analysis of case-controlled studies in 1889 children from six countries, forced expiratory volume in 1 second (FEV1) % predicted ($p < 0.00001$) and FVC% predicted ($p < 0.00001$) were significantly lower than controls; while FEV1/FVC ratio, total lung capacity (TLC) % predicted, and carbon monoxide diffusing capacity of the lungs (DLCO) were not significantly different than controls. Pooled analysis also supported the worsening of pulmonary function with recurrent episodes of ACS [14]. Inflammation in ACS has been associated with lung function deficits. Analysis of data from children in a 2-year randomized control study to examine the effects of vitamin D on SCD found a significant decline in FEV1 ($p = 0.015$) and FEF 25–75 ($p = 0.039$), in patients with a history of ACS. IP-10 level, a marker of TH-1 inflammation, was negatively correlated with changes in FVC in ACS patients, suggesting a role of interferon gamma-inducible chemokine receptors with lung function change. In patients with ACS, elevated levels of Th-2 inflammatory markers (IL-4, IL-5, IL-13) and IL-6 (a marker of monocyte inflammation) were found to have a negative influence on FVC and FEV1 [6]. Investigators have emphasized the role of vascular factors on obstructive airway phenotypes in SCD. In a study of 25 children with HbSS and 25 age- and ethnic-matched controls, children with SCD had greater pulmonary capillary blood volume ($p < 0.0001$) and increased respiratory system resistance (R5% predicted, $p = 0.0046$, as measured by impulse oscillometry) compared to controls. Among the children with HbSS, pulmonary capillary blood volume was positively correlated with R5% pred and the ratio of residual volume/total lung capacity (RV/TLC) and was negatively correlated with FEV1 and FEF 25–75, suggesting that increased resistance leading to airway obstruction in SCD may be related to increased cardiac output and increased pulmonary blood volume in response to chronic anemia [16].

More sensitive pulmonary function measurements may detect pulmonary function abnormalities earlier than spirometry or plethysmography. A recent study compared lung clearance index (LCI), a measure of ventilatory heterogeneity derived from a multiple breath washout technique, to changes in spirometry and body plethysmography in children with SCD versus controls. LCI ($p = 0.0001$), intra-acinar ventilation inhomogeneity (S_{acin}) ($p = 0.04$), z-scores for FEV1 ($p = 0.002$), FVC ($p = 0.002$), and TLC ($p = 0.002$) but not FEV1/FVC were significantly lower in SCD patients compared to controls. More patients (29%) had LCI >95th percentile of control subjects compared to patients with abnormal spirometry (23% had FEV1 < 5th percentile of the reference population). Significant differences from control subjects in LCI and S_{acin} but not in conductive ventilation inhomogeneity, (S_{cond}) and normal FEV1/FVC ratio suggest that the lung function changes were due to patchy peripheral lung disease. The multiple breath washout technique may serve as an early marker of peripheral lung disease before abnormalities in spirometry and plethysmography are detected [17].

Longitudinal cohort studies on children with SCD reveal a variable and inconsistent rate of decline in pulmonary function over time. A single-center longitudinal study in 312 children with SCD found an average decline in FEV1: 2.93% predicted per year for males, 2.95% predicted per year for females; average decline in TLC was 2.15% predicted per year in males, 2.43% predicted per year for females. Although only 18% of children had abnormal lung function at 17 years of age, the predominant change from 8 years of age was an increase in the number of children with a restrictive pattern (2.6% at age 8 vs. 18.7% at age 17 years) [18]. A longitudinal study of two cohorts of SCD patients compared to controls revealed a 0.93% decline in FEV1 over a 10-year follow-up. A younger cohort with a higher incidence of ACS episodes had a greater decline in FEV1 (1.45%) over a 2-year period and proportionately more children developed restrictive defects over time [13].

Treatment with disease modifiers may attenuate pulmonary function decline. A retrospective chart review of 62 children with SCD treated with hydroxyurea (HU) followed from 2000 to 2017 compared their spirometry to that of a group of untreated controls. FVC significantly increased in HU-treated children, while it decreased in controls (7.2 ± 17.1 vs. -3.4 ± 18.2, $p < 0.01$). HU is a disease modifier in SCD, resulting in increased fetal hemoglobin and decreased episodes of hemolysis [19].

Although universal screening for pulmonary function abnormalities is not recommended by the National Heart, Lung, and Blood Institute (NHLBI) or the American Society of Hematology (ASH) for asymptomatic patients with SCD, it should be considered in children with symptoms of cough, wheezing, shortness of breath, and oxygen desaturation. Results should be interpreted, and patients managed based on the presence of underlying complications associated with SCD, such as sleep-disordered breathing, asthma/wheezing, and/or pulmonary hypertension [5].

4. Asthma and airway hyperresponsiveness

Prevalence of asthma in non-Hispanic black children in the USA was reported to be 12.6% in 2017 by the Centers for Disease Control (CDC) [20]. Asthma is considered a distinct comorbidity in SCD and is associated with the higher rates of ACS, vaso-occlusive/pain crises, and mortality [1, 5, 21, 22]. The reported prevalence of asthma in children with SCD ranges from 8 to 53%, with several studies reporting a higher incidence of asthma in SCD compared to African American children. Differences in reported prevalence vary based on the definition of asthma, such as parental report of asthma, physician diagnosis of asthma, or use of an asthma medication [5, 15, 21, 22]. Multivariate logistic regression analysis of patients in the SAC cohort revealed that the presence of a parent with asthma ($p = 0.006$), wheezing causing shortness of breath, and/or wheezing with exercise ($p = .0001$) was 100% sensitive in identifying SCD children with asthma (physician-diagnosed asthma requiring asthma medications) [23].

Asthma and SCD have common inflammatory pathways. Diagnosing asthma in SCD patients is challenging since symptoms of cough, wheezing, shortness of breath, and chest pain, which are consistent with asthma, may also occur with chronic pulmonary inflammation, vasculopathy, and hemolysis in patients with SCD. The hallmarks of asthma pathophysiology, airway obstruction, and airway hyperreactivity from airway inflammation may be found in SCD patients, independent of an asthma diagnosis. Elevated serum IgE and leukotriene levels may also be found in SCD patients who have not been diagnosed with asthma [5, 24, 25]. SCD patients have elevated serum IgE levels, a biomarker of allergic asthma. Serum IgE elevation may be secondary to nonspecific immune activation of TH-2 pathways after ischemia-reperfusion injury in the lung in SCD, leading to an increased risk for asthma [21, 23, 24]. Cysteinyl leukotriene levels are elevated in SCD patients at baseline and during acute pain and ACS episodes. They are most elevated in patients with physician-diagnosed asthma and may contribute to the pathogenesis of vaso-occlusive disease [25]. Asthma is more common in SCD patients with allergies than in those without. Forty-five percent of children and adolescents in the SAC with a physician diagnosis of asthma had at least two positive skin prick tests for common aeroallergens compared to only 15% in those without asthma [23]. Although the prevalence of atopy in SCD is similar to that of the general population, reactivity to environmental allergens has been associated with increased incidence of ACS, independent of asthma diagnosis [21, 23]. Endothelial activation is considered the major pathway by which sickled red blood cells (RBCs) contribute to vaso-occlusion and consequently increased levels of pro-inflammatory cytokines, such as IL-3, granulocyte-macrophage colony-stimulating factor (GM-CSF), prostaglandin 2 (PGE-2), tumor necrosis factor alpha (TNF-α), and IL-6. The heightened inflammation is associated with pulmonary function abnormalities and susceptibility to infection. Heightened TH-2 inflammation has also been demonstrated in SCD mice models sensitized to ovalbumin. Arginine deficiency is a common pathophysiologic feature of allergic asthma and SCD. In SCD, increased hemolysis of red cells leads to low arginine bioavailability and is associated with complications, such as pulmonary hypertension and vaso-occlusive pain episodes. In asthma associated with SCD, increased arginase released by hemolysis and increased pulmonary eosinophilic inflammation decreasing arginine uptake may have an additive effect [26].

Wheezing has been reported in 26% of SCD patients with ACS and may be a marker of SCD severity [24]. In a retrospective cohort study of 262 patients with SCD who presented to an urban emergency department over a 4-year period, 19% had at least one presentation in which wheezing was documented, although less than 50% underwent an asthma diagnosis. Wheezing on physical examination was associated with more than twice the incidence of vaso-occlusive crises and ACS episodes, independent of an asthma diagnosis [27].

Airway hyperresponsiveness has been demonstrated in 17–77% of SCD patients and signifies airway lability secondary to bronchial inflammation [21, 24]. Leong was the first to describe airway hyperresponsiveness by cold air challenge or bronchodilator administration in 64% of SCD patients, independent of an asthma diagnosis [28, 29]. Lactate dehydrogenase (LDH) is a marker of hemolysis and has been associated with hyperresponsiveness to methacholine, suggesting that chronic hemolysis leads to inflammation in SCD, independent of a diagnosis of asthma [21, 24].

A diagnosis of asthma has been associated with increased disease-related morbidity in children with SCD. It is postulated that: (1) asthmatic bronchoconstriction-induced ventilation-perfusion mismatch leads to local tissue hypoxia and subsequent red blood cell sickling and/or (2) increased inflammation from oxidative stress and increased endothelial adhesion molecule expression and vaso-occlusion trigger the cascade of pathophysiologic events leading to respiratory complications in SCD [3, 30]. A pooled analysis of three different cohorts of children with SCD, that is, Cooperative Study of Sickle Cell Disease (CSSCD), Silent Cerebral Infarct Transfusion (SIT), and SAC, resulted in a dataset of 1685 participants, a mean follow-up of 6.1 years, and a total of 10,216 patient years with 23.1% diagnosed with asthma. Using negative binomial regression, with covariates of sex, age, hemoglobin, and white blood cell count, a significant positive association was found between asthma diagnosis and pain (IRR = 1.34, $p < 0.001$) and ACS episodes (IRR = 1.89, $p < 0.001$) [21].

SCD patients should be screened for recurrent respiratory symptoms, including wheezing, shortness of breath, exercise limitation, a personal history of allergies/atopy, and a family history of asthma, particularly a parental history of asthma [5, 24]. A validated asthma screening tool such as the Breathmobile questionnaire was found to have 87% sensitivity and 85% specificity in detecting a clinical diagnosis of asthma in school-aged children with SCD [31]. Referral to a pulmonary specialist should also be considered in patients with two or more episodes of ACS, the first episode of ACS in a child <4 years of age, life-threatening episode of ACS requiring RBC exchange transfusion, and concerns for sleep-disordered breathing [29]. Positive screening warrants further evaluation and management, including pulmonary function testing, which may reveal reversible airway obstruction supporting an asthma diagnosis and/or allergy testing if symptoms suggest that sensitization to environmental allergens are exacerbating symptoms [5, 15, 24, 30, 32].

Treatment of the SCD patient with asthma includes optimization of SCD management with the use of disease modifying therapy such as hydroxyurea, which has been shown to reduce morbidity and mortality [24]. When the diagnosis of persistent asthma is suggested by history (repeated wheezing and cough with a bronchodilator response, and personal and family history of atopy and asthma in a first-degree relative), therapy is based on NHLBI and GINA (Global Initiative for Asthma) guidelines [24]. The mainstay of therapy for patients with persistent disease includes anti-inflammatory controllers such as inhaled corticosteroids (ICS) alone or in combination with long-acting bronchodilators (LABA) and leukotriene receptor antagonists. Oral steroids, which are usually used to treat asthma exacerbations, carry a risk for acute vaso-occlusive pain and hospital readmission in SCD patients and should be used cautiously. Inhaled corticosteroids have not been associated with increased vaso-occlusive risk. While leukotriene receptor antagonists may have a role specifically in the treatment of asthma and SCD, they are associated with increased behavioral side effects compared to ICS [5, 21, 24, 30]. Further understanding of the inflammatory pathways in SCD may help to determine more effective treatments specific to this disorder.

5. Sleep-disordered breathing

The spectrum of sleep-disordered breathing (SDB) encompasses obstructive sleep apnea (OSA), central sleep apnea (CSA), and sleep-related hypoventilation, which in combination with hypoxemia may significantly impact patients with SCD [4]. Though the underlying mechanisms are not clearly understood, it has been suggested that children with SCD are at increased risk for SDB, with an estimated prevalence of around 36% [32]. Children with SCD are at increased risk for OSA because of compensatory lymphoid hyperplasia and subsequent adenotonsillar hypertrophy following splenic infarction; however, the mechanisms behind CSA or sleep-related hypoventilation are less clear. In adults, CSA may be more prevalent because of chronic opioid use and comorbid congestive heart failure [4]. Sleep architecture and sleep efficiency may be disrupted because of SCD-associated pain, particularly that of VOE. Shapiro et al. found that in children with increased SCD-associated pain, both sleep duration and sleep quality decreased [33]. The reciprocal relationship, in which children with poor sleep quality are at increased risk for pain [34], has also been shown. This is in addition to data that have shown that nocturnal oxyhemoglobin desaturations and nocturnal hypoxemia are prevalent in children with SCD (40%) and are associated with increased VOE [35].

Screening for SDB starts with a comprehensive sleep history and may be further strengthened with validated screening tools, such as the Sleep-Related Breathing Disorder scale, a component of the Pediatric Sleep Questionnaire (PSQ-SRBD) [36]. The gold standard for diagnosis of SDB is polysomnography (PSG); however, ASH does not recommend universal screening for SDB with PSG in asymptomatic children with SCD [34]. Instead, ASH recommends in-laboratory PSG for children who present with snoring, witnessed apneas, obesity, excessive daytime sleepiness, unexplained daytime or nocturnal hypoxemia, and a history of pulmonary hypertension. While traditional risk factors for SDB, especially OSA, may be absent in patients with SCD, the optimal time for screening is unclear and further objective testing is necessary. A 2020 prospective cohort study utilized the I'M SLEEPY sleep apnea questionnaire, previously validated in pediatrics, to screen for SDB in 100 children with SCD [34, 35]. Nineteen patients had a positive screen and were referred for PSG, of whom ten completed a PSG and seven had OSA. The most common responses included snoring, difficulty concentrating, and excessive daytime fatigue. The sensitivity and negative predicative values of this screen were 82 and 85%, respectively.

OSA is the result of recurrent upper airway obstruction and results in fragmented sleep and intermittent hypoxemia [37]. Among the general population in the United States, it is prevalent in 1–5% of children; however, it is thought that OSA may be more prevalent among those with SCD with reported prevalence between 5 and 79% [37]. Feld et al. retrospectively evaluated a cohort of children with both SCD and asthma who underwent PSG and reported an OSA prevalence of 59% that was also associated with both a lower nocturnal oxygen saturation nadir and a lower median daytime oxygen saturation [38]. In the SAC study, Rosen et al. identified an OSA prevalence between 10% (with an obstructive apnea-hypopnea index (OAHI) cutoff of ≥5 events/hr) and 41% (with an OAHI cutoff of ≥1 event/hr) among 243 children (median age 10 years), most of whom had HbSS [37]. There appears to be some variability in OSA classification, with the SAC study reporting predominantly mild OSA compared to a higher percentage of severe OSA reported in other studies [39].

OSA may affect other common SCD comorbidities. Feld et al. looked at the effect of OSA on clinical outcomes in children with SCD and found that, regardless of OSA, there was no difference in reported asthma severity [38]. Katz et al. performed a retrospective review of nearly 650 children with SCD who underwent screening for OSA over an 11-year period and compared SCD-associated complications in those with OSA (n = 136) to a matched-control set of children without OSA [40]. This study described an increase in the rate of SCD complications, notably hospitalizations for both ACS and pneumonia. Neurocognitive complications are described in both OSA and SCD; however, the association between OSA and SCD with respect to neurocognitive complications is less understood [41]. A retrospective cohort study, utilizing the US Representative Kids' Inpatient Database (KID), found that among 204,000 pediatric hospital discharges for SCD during the study period covering 15 years, < 2% carried a diagnosis of OSA. Those with OSA were more likely to have neurological complications (3.45 vs. 2.17%, p = 0.0014), particularly seizures (2.91 vs. 1.66%, p = 0.0003), and were more likely to have ACS (11.27 vs. 8.85%, p = 0.003) [42].

Since upper airway lymphoid tissue hypertrophy is the most common cause of OSA in children, the American Academy of Pediatrics recommends adenotonsillectomy (tonsillectomy and adenoidectomy (T&A)) as the preferred and first-line treatment for OSA [43]. Complications following T&A among the general population include postoperative hemorrhage and pulmonary edema, velopharyngeal insufficiency, and nerve palsy [44]. Though the benefits of T&A in children without underlying SCD have been studied previously, the extent to which T&A provides improvement in symptoms related to OSA in patients with SCD is less clear. Farrell et al. recently performed a retrospective review of 132 children ($\leq$ 18 years of age) with SCD (the majority of whom have HbSS disease) who underwent T&A for OSA as diagnosed on PSG [45]. This study found a significant improvement in several PSG parameters postoperatively, including a lower mean apnea-hypopnea index (7.6 versus 1.3 events/hour, $p = 0.0001$), higher mean oxygen nadir (81.2 versus 89.3%, $p = 0.0003$), and a higher mean oxygen saturation (95.7 versus 97%, $p = 0.016$). Complications occurred in 11.4% of the population, with the most common complication being postoperative ACS. While the review of this cohort 12 months after T&A showed a significant decrease in the mean number of emergency department visits, there was no significant change in the frequency of VOE or ACS. A similar study by Liguoro et al. looked at postoperative data from a small cohort of children with SCD, 19 patients in total, who underwent T&A and found that though there were improvements in PSG parameters, including mean oxygen nadir as well as a decreased mean annual rate of ACS; there was no change in the incidence of VOE or hospitalization rates [46]. Based on these studies, it seems apparent that T&A is beneficial in patients with SCD with respect to OSA; however, long-term implications with respect to SCD-related morbidity (i.e., ACS, VOE) are less clear. The impact that hydroxyurea may have on OSA in children is less well established. A 2017 chart review focused on two children with OSA, one of whom had concurrent HbSS disease and the other HbSβ° thalassemia, who had shown both improvement in symptoms and resolution in OSA confirmed on PSG approximately 1 year after initiation of hydroxyurea [47]. Whether well-established therapies such as hydroxyurea or newer medical therapies, including crizanlizumab and voxelotor, are viable treatments for patients with concurrent SCD and OSA is yet to be determined.

6. Thromboembolism

Venous thromboembolism (VTE) and pulmonary embolism affect 25% of adults with SCD and carry increased risk for mortality but are not common in children [1]. A retrospective observational study of 1062 patients revealed an incidence of 0.2% primarily in children with central venous lines (CVLs) over a 12-year period [48]. Using the Pediatric Health Information System (PHIS) database with data from 48 participating US institutions from 2009 to 2015, 1.7% of patients developed a VTE. The median age at diagnosis was 15.9 years. CVL placement, chronic renal disease, history of stroke, female sex, length of hospitalization, intensive care unit (ICU) utilization, and older age were significantly associated with VTE [49]. VTE is often overlooked in SCD because limb pain is attributed to VOE or chest pain to ACS. *In situ* microvascular thrombosis occurs in these patients and large vessel thrombi may not be seen, unless specialized tests are ordered [1, 4].

All three aspects of Virchow's triad (hypercoagulability, endothelial dysfunction, and hemostasis) create a thrombogenic environment in SCD. Patients with SCD have both traditional and SCD-specific risks for hypercoagulability and thrombus formation [1]. Traditional risk factors include frequent hospitalization and immobilization, use of CVL for red cell exchange or chronic transfusion therapy, need for orthopedic surgery for avascular necrosis of the hip or shoulder, cholecystectomy, splenectomy, and increased pregnancy-related VTE. SCD-related risk factors for VTE include impaired fibrinolysis and upregulation of cellular adhesion molecules. Alteration in sickled red cell structure leads to intravascular hemolysis and externalization of highly procoagulant phosphatidylserine on the red cell membrane. The sickled red cells are more adhesive to the endothelium and the capture of adhesive red cells, leukocytes, and platelets to the endothelial wall triggers vaso-occlusion [1]. SCD patients have dysregulation of factors that initiate and perpetuate hemostasis, as evidenced by decreased levels of natural coagulants, such as protein C, protein S, antithrombin III (ATIII), factors V, VI, IX, and XII. SCD patients have increased circulating levels of antiphospholipid antibodies, and elevated plasma levels of thrombin-antithrombin complexes and prothrombin fragment 1 + 2 (a marker of thrombin and fibrin generation as well as platelet activation). During vaso-occlusive crises, increased tissue factor expression, increased circulating fibrinogen, von Willebrand factor, and clotting factors VII and VIII may predispose patients to VTE. Pulmonary emboli (PE) have also been associated with ACS episodes [4].

A study of 22,631 children with SCD (median age 10.8 years (range: <0.1–20.9)) utilizing the PHIS database from January 2010 to June 2021 revealed a prevalence of hospitalization for PE of 0.3%. The median age was 17.4 years (range: 6.6–20.9 yrs.) at PE diagnosis. Patients with PE had longer hospitalization and more frequent intensive care unit admissions than patients without PE ($p < 0.001$). Risk factors significantly associated with PE on multivariable analysis included older age, history of CVL, ACS, and exchange transfusion. Mortality was not significantly different between those with and without PE [50].

The d-Dimer test has limited predictive value in diagnosing PE associated with SCD since it may be elevated due to the chronic activation of the coagulation cascade. Current guidelines recommend a compression Doppler for patients suspected of having lower extremity deep venous thromboses (DVTs). Ventilation-perfusion scans may identify PE. Computed tomography pulmonary angiography (CTPA) is currently the test of choice for suspected PE [1, 3].

While anticoagulants are usually prescribed for adults with ACS, children are not routinely given anticoagulants, unless a diagnosis of embolism is made. Anticoagulant prophylaxis in children is reserved for those with additional thrombosis risk, aside from SCD. Antithrombotic therapy for proximal DVT or PE follows 2016 American College of Chest Physician and 2018 ASH guidelines for the treatment of pediatric venous thromboembolism with 3–6 months of anticoagulation [1, 3, 4, 51, 52]. For patients with SCD-PH and VTE, indefinite anticoagulation may be considered in patients without a significant bleeding risk. Duration of therapy may be altered based on clinical status, for example, resolution of VTE on imaging, bleeding risk, or recurrence of VTE [1, 34].

7. Ventricular dysfunction

Sickle cell anemia has a profound impact on the cardiac anatomy and function in children with SCD. Cardiac dilation is well recognized in young children with SCD [53–56], with dilation leading to eccentric left ventricular hypertrophy. In addition, the left ventricle (LV) can develop both systolic and diastolic dysfunctions in children with sickle cell anemia, with diastolic dysfunction being much more common than systolic dysfunction.

Cardiac dilation occurs in sickle cell anemia due to the state of chronic anemia, increased blood volume, and stroke volume [53, 57]. It has been found that the increased cardiac output in patients with SCD occurs due to this increased stroke volume, with a comparatively minimal increase in heart rate [53]. LV wall stress is directly increased by LV afterload and radius of the LV, and inversely related to wall thickness. As the radius of the LV increases with cardiac dilation, so does the LV wall stress. To compensate for this, the wall thickness increases, mostly to a degree to keep the LV wall thickness normal to mildly increased, which leads to eccentric hypertrophy [58]. Studies on children with SCD have shown that the majority (50–60%) of children have dilation of the left heart, with a smaller percentage (20%) having increased LV wall thickness, with left heart abnormalities correlating with severity of anemia [54, 59].

Systolic dysfunction of the left ventricle is not common in children with SCD. The prevalence of pediatric patients with decreased systolic function indicated by a decreased shortening fraction (SF) and ejection fraction (EF) is very low, ranging from 0 to 5% [54, 55, 59, 60]. In adults, the prevalence of systolic dysfunction is only 9% [61]. SF and EF are LV function measurements highly influenced by preload, afterload, and heart rate; therefore, analyses of patients with SCD with these measures may not represent the heart's actual contractility. Some more recent studies have analyzed LV contractility and systolic function using load-independent measurements and have found differing results. Some have shown LV contractility to be preserved [56], whereas others found a decrease in contractility [62]. The use of speckle tracking echocardiography can be used to identify abnormalities of LV "twist" in systole, with the normal LV having clockwise rotation at the base and counterclockwise rotation at the apex in systole. In a study performed by Di Maria et al., the basal LV rotation in systole was significantly lower in children with SCD [63]. In adults and adolescents, Braga et al. found that patients with SCD had significantly decreased twist (sum of basal clockwise rotation and apical counterclockwise rotation) in comparison with normal controls [64].

Both invasive and noninvasive measures of LV diastolic function in adults with sickle cell anemia have shown a high prevalence of LV diastolic dysfunction (DD). Cardiac catheterization performed on adults with pulmonary hypertension (PH) shows that ~50% also have DD [65]. Other studies have demonstrated a 65% prevalence of DD in adults with SCD and PH, and 20% in those without PH [66]. Using Doppler echocardiography assessment in adults, Sachdev et al. found that 18% of patients had diastolic dysfunction (defined as mitral inflow $E/A < 1$, where the E/A ratio denotes the ratio of the early (E) to late (A) ventricular filling velocities) and this group had higher risk of mortality with a risk ratio of 3.5. This study also found a further increased risk of mortality with DD and PH with a risk ratio for death of 12 [61]. There is a growing collection of research on pediatric patients with SCD and the assessment of LV DD. Zilberman et al. demonstrated that echocardiogram (echo) markers of LV stiffness, the E/E' ratios, were significantly higher in pediatric patients with SCD [67]. In 54% of pediatric patients with SCD, echo findings of elevated LV filling pressures (with septal $E/E' > 8$) were identified by Olson et al. [68]. Alsaied et al. studied adults and children (age range 8–43 years, mean 21) with SCD and found a 30% prevalence of DD, which was associated with decreased exercise capacity [69].

Hankins et al. evaluated children with SCD and iron overload; 77% had low E' (mean mitral annular velocity), and all had elevated E/E', both measures indicating diastolic dysfunction; there was no correlation with diastolic dysfunction and iron deposition in the heart [70]. Johnson et al. studied children with SCD and found increased E/E' ratios, and greater diastolic dysfunction was found in those with sleeping and awake oxygen desaturations [71].

More recent research utilizing speckle tracking echocardiography and cardiac magnetic resonance imaging (cMRI) has provided further insights into the cause of this diastolic dysfunction. As noted previously, the use of speckle tracking echocardiography can be used to identify abnormalities of LV "twist" in systole, as well as the "untwisting" in diastole. In a study by Di Maria et al., the peak untwisting rate was significantly lower in children with SCD [63]. Other newer methods of assessing diastolic dysfunction include assessing left atrial (LA) strain with speckle tracking. Jhaveri et al. studied children with SCD and found a significant reduction in LA strain that correlated with the degree in decreased hemoglobin—for every decrease of 1 g/dL of hemoglobin, there was decrease in LA strain by 3.2% [72].

Using cMRI along with echocardiogram findings, Desai et al. compared adults with SCD with normal controls and found that patients with SCD had an increased incidence of myocardial fibrosis, abnormal myocardial perfusion reserve index (both by cMRI), and DD (by echocardiogram), with 29% of patients having DD. The DD did not correlate with cardiac iron overload [73]. Niss et al. studied adults and children with SCD; 29% met echo criteria for DD and 42% had diastolic abnormalities that did not reach the threshold for DD. Patients with DD had a greater prevalence of diffuse myocardial fibrosis on magnetic resonance imaging (MRI) (measured by quantifying the myocardial extracellular volume fraction, ECV). Greater ECV was associated with statistically significantly higher N-terminal pro hormone B-type brain natriuretic peptide (NT-proBNP) levels and correlated with the degree of anemia [74]. Alsaied & Niss et al. demonstrated that left atrial (LA) dysfunction (as measured by LA stiffness), and therefore, LV diastolic dysfunction were related to diffuse myocardial fibrosis (again by MRI ECV), exercise impairment, and increased tricuspid regurgitation velocities (TRVs) [69, 74].

8. Pulmonary hypertension

Pulmonary hypertension (PH) is a leading cause of morbidity and mortality in adults with SCD [75]. PH is defined as a resting mean pulmonary artery pressure (PAP) over 20 mm Hg measured by right heart catheterization (RHC). Hemodynamically, PH is subdivided as precapillary PH if the pulmonary capillary wedge pressure (PCWP) or left ventricular end-diastolic pressure (LVEDP) at right heart catheterization is ≤15 mm Hg and as postcapillary PH if the PCWP or LVEDP is >15 mm Hg. About half of SCD-related PH patients have precapillary PH with potential etiologies of (1) a nitric oxide (NO) deficiency state and vasculopathy, consequent to intravascular hemolysis, (2) chronic pulmonary thromboembolism, or (3) upregulated hypoxic responses secondary to anemia, low oxygen (O_2) saturation, and microvascular obstruction [53, 76]. The remainder have postcapillary PH secondary to left ventricular dysfunction, which is common in patients with SCD, possibly related to ventricular dilation and concentric hypertrophy of the myocardium as a response to chronic anemia and relative systemic hypertension [75].

The initial test of choice to screen for PH is transthoracic echocardiography (TTE). In general, the tricuspid regurgitation velocity (TRV) measured during TTE with estimated right atrial pressure is considered a valid estimate of systolic PAP. Other signs of PH on TTE include right ventricular hypertrophy and/or dilation, systolic flattening of the interventricular septum, right atrial dilation, and increasing tricuspid regurgitation (TR). Once PH is diagnosed, further evaluation is needed to identify contributors to PH that might require focused treatment, such as hypoxemia due to sleep-disordered breathing including obstructive sleep apnea (OSA), venous thromboembolism, or portal hypertension. Because of the known association of OSA with PH in non-SCD populations, the clinical guidelines for diagnosis of PH in SCD recommend a formal sleep study for all SCD patients with an elevated TRV [77]. In addition, the evaluation for other contributors to PH typically includes laboratory testing (liver function tests, antinuclear antibody), pulmonary function testing, radionuclide ventilation-perfusion scan, and CTPA.

N-terminal-pro-hormone B-type brain natriuretic peptide (NT-proBNP) has been evaluated as potential screening tool for PH in the pediatric SCD population [78, 79]. In adults with SCD, the degree of NT-proBNP elevation correlated with mortality [80]. The cutoff level for NT-proBNP is not defined in children, although guidelines suggest NT-proBNP >160 pg./mL to be indicative of an elevated PAP. A retrospective study of children with SCD found a higher median NT-proBNP of 70 pg./mL in 8–14-year-olds than age-matched controls. NT-proBNP levels were associated with markers of hemolysis, that is, reticulocyte count ($r = .25$, $p = 0.01$) and LDH $r = .47$, p.001). A positive correlation was found between NT-proBNP and diastolic left ventricular size ($r = 0.28$, $p = 0.047$) [81]. Hence, NT-proBNP and TTE as noninvasive tools may play a role in identifying PH, prior to RHC. Of note, NT-proBNP measurements may be misleading in patients with renal insufficiency or left heart failure [77].

The reported prevalence of PH in the pediatric age group with SCD varies, with studies including older patient populations reporting a higher prevalence suggesting a disease progression from childhood into adulthood secondary to chronic hemolysis and systemic vasculopathy [82]. An analysis of pediatric studies combining almost 1200 children revealed a prevalence of elevated TRV (>2.5 m/s) in 25%, while moderate to severely elevated TRV (>3.0 m/s) was noted in 4% of children [83]. Children with more severe hemolysis, anemia, and acute chest episodes are at a higher risk for developing PH.

Universal screening for PH is not recommended by the NHLBI and ASH for asymptomatic patients with SCD. A screening for TTE is recommended in children with symptoms suggestive of PH (e.g., exercise intolerance, fatigue, peripheral edema, and chest pain) [84]. The American Thoracic Society (ATS) suggests a one-time TTE in asymptomatic children with SCD who are aged 8 to 18 years (sooner in those with severe hemolytic anemia) [85]. If the TRV is elevated (>2.5 m/s), the patient may require additional evaluation starting with an RHC. Once individuals with SCD reach adulthood (18 years of age), TTE is recommended every 1 to 3 years, using the shorter intervals for those with respiratory symptoms, TRV ≥2.5 m/sec on prior echocardiogram, greater frequency of pain episodes, prior thromboembolic events, or greater severity of hemolytic anemia [77].

A general approach to the management of SCD-related PH involves supportive care, use of SCD-specific therapies, and consideration of specific agents for PH. Examples of supportive care and treatment of comorbidities include oxygen therapy for those with low oxygen saturation, treatment of left ventricular failure in those with postcapillary PH, and anticoagulation for those with thromboembolism. SCD-specific treatments, such as hydroxyurea or chronic transfusion therapy, may be of benefit by raising the hemoglobin concentration, reducing hemolysis, and preventing vaso-occlusive events that cause additional increases in PAP. A recent study by Dhar et al. found that hydroxyurea therapy was associated with a decrease in TRV in children with SCD [55]. Another prospective study of 204 children with SCD found that hydroxyurea use was associated with an estimated 5% decline in TRV after 2 years [86]. A carefully selected subgroup of symptomatic patients with RHC-confirmed elevation in pulmonary vascular resistance (PVR) and normal PCWP should be referred to an expert in PH for close follow-up and consideration whether PH-targeted therapy should be attempted. Specific therapies for the treatment of PH include prostacyclin derivatives, endothelin receptor antagonists, and phosphodiesterase-5 inhibitors [87]. Bosentan, an endothelin receptor blocker, appeared to be well tolerated in a randomized, double-blind, placebo-controlled trial of patients with SCD and PH, although the small sample size precluded an analysis of its efficacy [88]. Another randomized, double-blind, placebo-controlled study designed to evaluate the safety and efficacy of sildenafil was prematurely halted after interim analysis showed that sildenafil-treated patients were likely to have more acute sickle cell pain crises (35%) compared with placebo-treated patients (14%) [89]. Therefore, response to PH-targeted therapies appears to be different in this patient population.

In adults with SCD, PH is associated with increased mortality [90]. While PH is not associated with a higher mortality in children with SCD, these children may be at increased risk of cardiopulmonary decline [91]. A comprehensive assessment for symptoms suggestive of PH should be performed at each visit, and if suspected, evaluation should begin with a TTE. Currently, there is not enough evidence to suggest that early identification and treatment of children with SCD and elevated TRV improve survival. Treatment and follow-up of patients with confirmed PH should be performed at a center with experience in the treatment of pediatric PH, and this should occur in close conjunction with the hematology team.

8.1 Therapy

Treatment options for sickle cell disease include disease modifying treatments such as hydroxyurea, voxelotor, crizanlizumab, and red blood cell transfusions as well as curative or transformative therapies such as bone marrow transplantation and newly approved gene therapies.

Blood transfusions are lifesaving for individuals living with SCD. There are several instances where transfusions may be administered. They can be used to treat or prevent acute and chronic complications. Acute complications for which transfusions are recommended include splenic sequestration crisis, stroke, acute chest syndrome, aplastic crisis, or multiorgan failure [92]. Transfusions are not routinely recommended for vaso-occlusive pain episodes, priapism, or avascular necrosis. Chronic transfusion therapy is usually reserved for primary or secondary prevention of stroke. Rarely, they are used in patients who continue to have recurrent episodes of vaso-occlusive pain and acute chest syndrome, despite being on hydroxyurea. It is important to consult with a sickle cell specialist if a blood transfusion is being considered as the volume to be given will need careful thought. Transfusion therapy may lead to immediate and/or delayed side effects including transfusion reactions—acute and delayed; increased viscosity, which may increase stroke risk; concern for fluid overload; iron overload; and alloimmunization. It is important to counsel families about these side effects so care may be sought immediately.

Hydroxyurea is the oldest Food and Drug Administration (FDA)-approved disease modifying treatment for individuals living with SCD. One of the main benefits of hydroxyurea is an increase in fetal hemoglobin, which prevents sickling. Additional benefits include improved RBC rheology and survival. The effects of hydroxyurea on SCD have been studied for several decades. It reduces and prevents vaso-occlusive episodes, including pain and acute chest syndrome, transfusion requirements, and inpatient admissions. It has been shown to decrease morbidity and mortality [93]. It can prevent strokes in individuals with abnormal transcranial Doppler velocities, who do not have severe vasculopathy [94]. It is safe to administer in young children [95]. Hydroxyurea may be started as early as 9 months of age in individuals with sickle cell anemia (HBSS, HbSβ° thalassemia) to prevent any complications [84]. Current studies about hydroxyurea are looking at personalized dosing options [96]. Hydroxyurea is very well tolerated; myelosuppression is a potential side effect that requires monitoring.

Voxelotor is a novel oral disease modifying treatment approved by the FDA for adults and pediatric patients 4 years of age and older with sickle cell disease. It decreases the polymerization of HbS, which is responsible for much of the pathophysiology in SCD. Voxelotor binds reversibly to the alpha-globin chain of Hb and increases its affinity for oxygen. It has been shown to increase baseline hemoglobin by >1 g/dL [97]. However, there are no current data thus far demonstrating reduction in the frequency of pain episodes [98]. It is generally well tolerated. The most common adverse reactions include headache and abdominal pain. They can interfere with measurement of hemoglobin subtypes *via* liquid chromatography, thus affecting laboratory interpretation of hemoglobin electrophoresis.

Crizanlizumab is an FDA-approved novel injectable therapeutic agent that is approved for adults and pediatric patients with SCD, regardless of genotype, aged 16 years and older. In vaso-occlusive episodes, there is significant upregulation of P-selectin on the endothelial cells and platelets. These cell-to-cell adhesions are responsible for the pathogenesis of sickle-related pain crisis in individuals with SCD [99]. Crizanlizumab is a humanized monoclonal antibody that binds to P-selectin and inhibits the interaction between P-selectin and glycoprotein ligand 1, thereby decreasing adhesion [99]. In a phase 2 randomized, placebo-controlled trial, high-dose crizanlizumab resulted in 35% reduction in pain-related episodes in participants taking hydroxyurea and 50% reduction in those not on hydroxyurea [99]. It is administered intravenously, starting every 2 weeks and then as monthly infusions. It is generally well tolerated and adverse effects include infusion reactions, arthralgia, diarrhea, pruritus, vomiting, and chest pain.

Hematopoietic stem cell transplantation (HSCT) has been utilized as a curative treatment for SCD for the past four decades. An analysis of 996 patients who underwent HSCT between 2008 and 2017 shows that best outcomes are achieved when the donor is a human leukocyte antigen (HLA)-match sibling and the HSCT is performed before 13 years of age [100]. All patients with stroke, abnormal transcranial Doppler velocities, frequent acute painful events, and recurrent acute chest syndrome should be offered HSCT as a treatment option [101]. The risks related to HSCT are graft rejection, graft-versus-host disease, infections, infertility, and death.

Many people living with sickle cell disease do not have HLA-match donor. Therefore, gene therapy using patient's own hematopoietic stem cells is an attractive alternative. There are three main approaches to gene therapy in sickle cell disease: (1) gene addition, (2) gene editing, and (3) gene correction. In LentiGlobin trials, patients' stem cells were transduced with a lentiviral vector encoding a modified β-globin gene, which resulted in the production of an antisickling hemoglobin, HbA^{T87Q98}. Thirty-five patients received treatment and engrafted. All of the 25 evaluable patients had complete resolution of severe vaso-occlusive events. Hemoglobin level increased from 8.5 to 11 gm/dl [101]. In another approach, CRISPR-Cas9

(Clustered regularly interspaced short palindromic repeats -CRISPR-associated protein 9) technology was used to target BCL11A (transcription factor B-cell lymphoma/leukemia 11A), a transcription factor that represses γ-globin expression and fetal hemoglobin [102]. One patient with transfusion-dependent thalassemia and one patient with sickle cell disease underwent this treatment, which resulted in pancellular distribution of HbF in red blood cells and led to transfusion independence in the thalassemia patient and resolution of pain crises in the sickle cell patient. The Food and Drug Administration (FDA) has approved both these treatments in December 2023 for patients with SCD ≥12 years with recurrent vaso-occlusive events.

9. Conclusion

Sickle cell disease (SCD) is characterized by hemolysis, increased endothelial adhesion, inflammation, and vasculopathy. Various cardiopulmonary complications may occur in children including ACS, pulmonary function abnormalities, asthma, sleep disordered breathing, ventricular dysfunction, thromboembolism, and pulmonary hypertension that may lead to more severe outcomes in adulthood. Repeated episodes of ACS may be associated with increased inflammation and decreased longitudinal lung function in children. Increased airway hyperresponsiveness, leukotriene levels, and airway inflammation are seen in SCD patients. Children with SCD are at increased risk for asthma, sleep-disordered breathing, and obstructive sleep apnea, which have been associated with an increase in the rate of SCD complications such as VOE or ACS. Diastolic dysfunction associated with chronic anemia in SCD patients has been associated with decreased exercise capacity. Evidence of pulmonary hypertension in children with SCD suggests a disease progression from childhood into adulthood, secondary to chronic hemolysis and systemic vasculopathy. While most guidelines do not recommend routine screening or testing for complications in children, patients with symptoms, such as increased incidence of VOE or ACS, wheezing, shortness of breath, sleep-disordered breathing, or hypoxemia, should be screened and followed by specialists preferably in a multidisciplinary setting. Disease modifying treatments such as hydroxyurea may attenuate some of the cardiopulmonary complications in SCD. More studies need to be done to assess the long-term effects of newer disease modifying and transformative therapies.

Conflict of interest

Dr. Banu Aygun receives research funding from Pfizer and Bluebird Bio. She has participated in advisory board meetings for Global Blood Therapeutics, Agios, Pfizer, and Bluebird Bio. Dr. Elizabeth Fiorino has served as a consultant for Boehringer Ingelheim, Simumetrix, and the France Foundation.

Author details

Maria Teresa Santiago[1,2,3]*, Lance Feld[1,2,3], Arushi Dhar[1,2,4], La Nyka Christian-Weekes[1,2,5], Abena Appiah-Kubi[1,2,5], Elizabeth Mitchell[1,2,4], Banu Aygun[1,2,5] and Elizabeth K. Fiorino[1,2,3]

1 Northwell, New Hyde Park, NY, The United States of America

2 Cohen Children's Medical Center, New Hyde Park, NY, The United States of America

3 Division of Pediatric Pulmonology, The United States of America

4 Division of Pediatric Cardiology, The United States of America

5 Division of Pediatric Hematology and Oncology and Cellular Therapy, The United States of America

*Address all correspondence to: msantiag@northwell.edu

References

[1] Pervaiz A, El-Baba F, Dhillon K, Daoud A, Soubani A. Pulmonary complications of sickle cell disease: A narrative clinical review. Advances in Respiratory Medicine. 2021;**89**(2):173-187. DOI: 10.5603/ARM.a2021.0011

[2] Piel FB, Hay SI, Gupta S, Weatherall DJ, Williams TN. Global burden of sickle cell anaemia in children under five, 2010-2050: Modelling based on demographics, excess mortality, and interventions. PLoS Medicine. 2013;**10**(7):e1001484. DOI: 10.1371/journal.pmed.1001484

[3] Mehari A, Klings ES. Chronic pulmonary complications of sickle cell disease. Chest. 2016;**149**(5):1313-1324. DOI: 10.1016/j.chest.2015.11.016

[4] Ruhl AP, Sadreameli SC, Allen JL, et al. Identifying clinical and research priorities in sickle cell lung disease. An official American Thoracic Society workshop report. Annals of the American Thoracic Society. 2019;**16**(9):e17-e32. DOI: 10.1513/AnnalsATS.201906-433RD

[5] Desai AA, Machado RF, Cohen RT. The cardiopulmonary complications of sickle cell disease. Hematology/Oncology Clinics of North America. 2022;**36**(6):1217-1237. DOI: 10.1016/j.hoc.2022.07.014

[6] De A, Williams S, Yao Y, Jin Z, Brittenham GM, Kattan M, et al. Acute chest syndrome, airway inflammation and lung function in sickle cell disease. PLoS One. 2023;**18**(3):e0283349. DOI: 10.1371/journal.pone.0283349

[7] Ploton MC, Sommet J, Koehl B, Gaschignard J, Holvoet L, Mariani-Kurkdjian P, et al. Respiratory pathogens and acute chest syndrome in children with sickle cell disease. Archives of Disease in Childhood. 2020;**105**(9):891-895. DOI: 10.1136/archdischild-2019-317315

[8] Assad Z, Michel M, Valtuille Z, Lazzati A, Boizeau P, Madhi F, et al. Incidence of acute chest syndrome in children with sickle cell disease following implementation of the 13-Valent pneumococcal conjugate vaccine in France. JAMA Network Open. 2022;**5**(8):e2225141. DOI: 10.1001/jamanetworkopen.2022.25141

[9] Almon P, Elenga N. How I treat acute chest syndrome in asthmatic children with sickle cell disease. A practical review. Hemoglobin. 2020;**44**(5):307-310. DOI: 10.1080/03630269.2020.1814321

[10] Koumbourlis AC, Hurlet-Jensen A, Bye MR. Lung function in infants with sickle cell disease. Pediatric Pulmonology. 1997;**24**(4):277-281. DOI: 10.1002/(sici)1099-0496(199710)24:4<277:aid-ppul6>3.0.co;2-h

[11] Arteta M, Campbell A, Nouraie M, Rana S, Onyekwere OC, Ensing G, et al. Abnormal pulmonary function and associated risk factors in children and adolescents with sickle cell anemia. Journal of Pediatric Hematology/Oncology. 2014;**36**(3):185-189. DOI: 10.1097/MPH.0000000000000011

[12] Ivankovich DT, Braga JAP, de Lanza FC, Solé D, Wandalsen GF. Lung function in infants with sickle cell anemia. The Journal of Pediatrics. 2019;**207**:252-254. DOI: 10.1016/j.jpeds.2018.11.036

[13] Lunt A, McGhee E, Sylvester K, Rafferty G, Dick M, Rees D, et al. Longitudinal assessment of lung function in children with sickle cell disease. Pediatric Pulmonology. 2016;**51**(7):717-723. DOI: 10.1002/ppul.23367

[14] Taksande A, Jameel PZ, Pujari D, Taksande B, Meshram R. Variation in pulmonary function tests among children with sickle cell anemia: A systematic review and meta-analysis. The Pan African Medical Journal. 2021;**39**:140. DOI: 10.11604/pamj.2021.39.140.28755

[15] Cohen RT, Strunk RC, Rodeghier M, Rosen CL, Kirkham FJ, Kirkby J, et al. Pattern of lung function is not associated with prior or future morbidity in children with sickle cell anemia. Annals of the American Thoracic Society. 2016;**13**(8):1314-1323. DOI: 10.1513/AnnalsATS.201510-706OC

[16] Wedderburn CJ, Rees D, Height S, Dick M, Rafferty GF, Lunt A, et al. Airways obstruction and pulmonary capillary blood volume in children with sickle cell disease. Pediatric Pulmonology. 2014;**49**(7):724. DOI: 10.1002/ppul.22952

[17] Arigliani M, Kirkham FJ, Sahota S, Riley M, Liguoro I, Castriotta L, et al. Lung clearance index may detect early peripheral lung disease in sickle cell anemia. Annals of the American Thoracic Society. 2022;**19**(9):1507-1515. DOI: 10.1513/AnnalsATS.202102-168OC

[18] MacLean JE, Atenafu E, Kirby-Allen M, MacLusky IB, Stephens D, Grasemann H, et al. Longitudinal decline in lung volume in a population of children with sickle cell disease. American Journal of Respiratory and Critical Care Medicine. 2008;**178**(10):1055-1059. DOI: 10.1164/rccm.200708-1219OC

[19] Kotwal N, Pillai DK, Darbari DS, Sun K, Koumbourlis AC. Spirometric changes after initiation of Hydroxyurea in children with sickle cell anemia. Journal of Pediatric Hematology/Oncology. 2022;**44**(6):e923-e925. DOI: 10.1097/MPH.0000000000000237

[20] Asthma. 2017 Archived National asthma data – Prevalence. 2017 [Internet] Available from: https://cdc.gov/asthma/archivedata/2017/2017_archived_national_data.html [Accessed: February 9, 2024]

[21] Willen SM, Rodeghier M, DeBaun MR. Asthma in children with sickle cell disease. Current Opinion in Pediatrics. 2019;**31**(3):349-356. DOI: 10.1097/MOP.0000000000000756

[22] Anim SO, Strunk RC, DeBaun MR. Asthma morbidity and treatment in children with sickle cell disease. Expert Review of Respiratory Medicine. 2011;**5**(5):635-645. DOI: 10.1586/ers.11.64

[23] Strunk RC, Cohen RT, Cooper BP, Rodeghier M, Kirkham FJ, Warner JO, et al. Wheezing symptoms and parental asthma are associated with a physician diagnosis of asthma in children with sickle cell anemia. The Journal of Pediatrics. 2014;**164**(4):821-826.e1. DOI: 10.1016/j.jpeds.2013.11.034

[24] Cohen RT, Klings ES, Strunk RC. Sickle cell disease: Wheeze or asthma? Asthma Research and Practice. 2015;**1**:14. DOI: 10.1186/s40733-015-0014-2

[25] Knight-Perry J, DeBaun MR, Strunk RC, Field JJ. Leukotriene pathway in sickle cell disease: A potential target for directed therapy. Expert Review of Hematology. 2009;**2**(1):57-68. DOI: 10.1586/17474086.2.1.57

[26] Samarasinghe AE, Rosch JW. Convergence of inflammatory pathways

in allergic asthma and sickle cell disease. Frontiers in Immunology. 2019;**10**:3058. DOI: 10.3389/fimmu.2019.03058

[27] Glassberg JA, Chow A, Wisnivesky J, Hoffman R, Debaun MR, Richardson LD. Wheezing and asthma are independent risk factors for increased sickle cell disease morbidity. British Journal of Haematology. 2012;**159**(4):472-479. DOI: 10.1111/bjh.12049

[28] Leong MA, Dampier C, Varlotta L, Allen JL. Airway hyperreactivity in children with sickle cell disease. The Journal of Pediatrics. 1997;**131**(2):278-283. DOI: 10.1016/s0022-3476(97)70166-5

[29] Boyd JH, Moinuddin A, Strunk RC, DeBaun MR. Asthma and acute chest in sickle-cell disease. Pediatric Pulmonology. 2004;**38**(3):229-232. DOI: 10.1002/ppul.20066

[30] Arigliani M, Gupta A. Management of chronic respiratory complications in children and adolescents with sickle cell disease. European Respiratory Review: An Official Journal of the European Respiratory Society. 2020;**29**(157):200054. DOI: 10.1183/16000617.0054-2020

[31] Sadreameli SC, Alade RO, Mogayzel PJ, McGrath-Morrow S, Strouse JJ. Asthma screening in pediatric sickle cell disease: A clinic-based program using questionnaires and spirometry. Pediatric Allergy, Immunology and Pulmonology. 2017;**30**(4):232-238. DOI: 10.1089/ped.2017.0776

[32] Caboot JB, Allen JL. Pulmonary complications of sickle cell disease in children. Current Opinion in Pediatrics. 2008;**20**(3):279-287. DOI: 10.1097/MOP.0b013e3282ff62c4

[33] Shapiro BS, Dinges DF, Orne EC, Bauer N, Reilly LB, Whitehouse WG, et al. Home management of sickle cell-related pain in children and adolescents: Natural history and impact on school attendance. Pain. 1995;**61**(1):139-144. DOI: 10.1016/0304-3959(94)00164-A

[34] Valrie CR, Gil KM, Redding-Lallinger R, Daeschner C. Brief report: Sleep in children with sickle cell disease: An analysis of daily diaries utilizing multilevel models. Journal of Pediatric Psychology. 2007;**32**(7):857-861. DOI: 10.1093/jpepsy/jsm016

[35] Needleman JP, Franco ME, Varlotta L, Reber-Brodecki D, Bauer N, Dampier C, et al. Mechanisms of nocturnal oxyhemoglobin desaturation in children and adolescents with sickle cell disease. Pediatric Pulmonology. 1999;**28**(6):418-422. DOI: 10.1002/(sici)1099-0496(199912)28:6<418::aid-ppul6>3.0.co;2-d

[36] Chervin RD, Hedger K, Dillon JE, Pituch KJ. Pediatric sleep questionnaire (PSQ): Validity and reliability of scales for sleep-disordered breathing, snoring, sleepiness, and behavioral problems. Sleep Medicine. 2000;**1**(1):21-32. DOI: 10.1016/s1389-9457(99)00009-x

[37] Rosen CL, Debaun MR, Strunk RC, Redline S, Seicean S, Craven DI, et al. Obstructive sleep apnea and sickle cell anemia. Pediatrics. 2014;**134**(2):273-281. DOI: 10.1542/peds.2013-4223. Epub 2014 Jul 14

[38] Feld L, Bhandari A, Allen J, Saxena S, Stefanovski D, Afolabi-Brown O. The impact of obstructive sleep apnea in children with sickle cell disease and asthma. Pediatric Pulmonology. 2023;**58**(11):3188-3194. DOI: 10.1002/ppul.26643

[39] Abijay CA, Kemper WC, Pham A, Johnson RF, Mitchell RB. Pediatric obstructive sleep Apnea and sickle cell disease: Demographic and polysomnographic features. The Laryngoscope. 2023;**133**(7):1766-1772. DOI: 10.1002/lary.30638

[40] Katz T, Schatz J, Roberts CW. Comorbid obstructive sleep apnea and increased risk for sickle cell disease morbidity. Sleep & Breathing = Schlaf & Atmung. 2018;**22**(3):797-804. DOI: 10.1007/s11325-018-1630-x

[41] Marcus CL, Brooks LJ, Draper KA, Gozal D, Halbower AC, Jones J, et al. Diagnosis and management of childhood obstructive sleep apnea syndrome. American Academy of Pediatrics. 2012;**130**(3):e714-e755. DOI: 10.1542/peds.2012-1672

[42] Tsou PY, Cielo CM, Xanthopoulos MS, Wang YH, Kuo PL, Tapia IE. The burden of obstructive sleep apnea in pediatric sickle cell disease: A kids' inpatient database study. Sleep. 2021;**44**(2):zsaa157. DOI: 10.1093/sleep/zsaa157

[43] Gozal D, Tan HL, Kheirandish-Gozal L. Treatment of obstructive sleep Apnea in children: Handling the unknown with precision. Journal of Clinical Medicine. 2020;**9**(3):888. DOI: 10.3390/jcm9030888

[44] Della Vecchia L, Passali FM, Coden E. Complications of adenotonsillectomy in pediatric age. Acta Bio-medica: Atenei Parmensis. 2020;**91**(1-S):48-53. DOI: 10.23750/abm.v91i1-S.9256

[45] Farrell AN, Goudy SL, Yee ME, Leu RM, Landry AM. Adenotonsillectomy in children with sickle cell disease and obstructive sleep apnea. International Journal of Pediatric Otorhinolaryngology. 2018;**111**:158-161. DOI: 10.1016/j.ijporl.2018.05.034

[46] Liguoro I, Arigliani M, Singh B, Van Geyzel L, Chakravorty S, Bossley C, et al. Beneficial effects of adenotonsillectomy in children with sickle cell disease. European Respiratory Journal Open Research. 2020;**6**(4):00071-02020. DOI: 10.1183/23120541.00071-2020

[47] Grady AJ, Hankins JS, Haberman B, Schoumacher R, Stocks RM. Hydroxyurea treatment effect on children with sickle cell disease and obstructive sleep apnea. Sleep & Breathing = Schlaf & Atmung. 2017;**21**(3):697-701. DOI: 10.1007/s11325-017-1458-9

[48] de Boechat TO, do Nascimento EM, de Lobo CLC, Ballas SK. Deep venous thrombosis in children with sickle cell disease. Pediatric Blood & Cancer. 2015;**62**(5):838-841. DOI: 10.1002/pbc.25431

[49] Kumar R, Stanek J, Creary S, Dunn A, O'Brien SH. Prevalence and risk factors for venous thromboembolism in children with sickle cell disease: An administrative database study. Blood Advances. 2018;**2**(3):285-291. DOI: 10.1182/bloodadvances.2017012336

[50] Bala N, Stanek J, Rodriguez V, Villella A. Prevalence and risk factors for pulmonary embolism in children with sickle cell disease: An institutional retrospective cohort study. Blood Coagulation & Fibrinolysis: An International Journal in Haemostasis and Thrombosis. 2023;**34**(5):289-294. DOI: 10.1097/MBC.0000000000001224

[51] Monagle P, Cuello CA, Augustine C, Bonduel M, Brandão LR, Capman T, et al. American Society of Hematology 2018 guidelines for management of venous thromboembolism: Treatment of pediatric venous thromboembolism. Blood Advances. 2018;**2**(22):3292-3316. DOI: 10.1182/bloodadvances.2018024786

[52] Ko RH, Thornburg CD. Venous thromboembolism in children with cancer and blood disorders. Frontiers in Pediatrics. 2017;**5**:12. DOI: 10.3389/fped.2017.00012

[53] Gladwin MT, Sachdev V. Cardiovascular abnormalities in sickle cell disease. Journal of the American College of Cardiology. 2012;**59**(13):1123-1133. DOI: 10.1016/j.jacc.2011.10.900

[54] Lester LA, Sodt PC, Hutcheon N, Arcilla RA. Cardiac abnormalities in children with sickle cell anemia. Chest. 1990;**98**(5):1169-1174. DOI: 10.1378/chest.98.5.1169

[55] Dhar A, Leung TM, Appiah-Kubi A, Gruber D, Aygun B, Serigano O, et al. Longitudinal analysis of cardiac abnormalities in pediatric patients with sickle cell anemia and effect of hydroxyurea therapy. Blood Advances. 2021;**5**(21):4406-4412. DOI: 10.1182/bloodadvances.2021005076

[56] Batra AS, Acherman RJ, Wong WY, Wood JC, Chan LS, Ramicone E, et al. Cardiac abnormalities in children with sickle cell anemia. American Journal of Hematology. 2002;**70**(4):306-312. DOI: 10.1002/ajh.10154

[57] Varat MA, Adolph RJ, Fowler NO. Cardiovascular effects of anemia. American Heart Journal. 1972;**83**(3):415-426. DOI: 10.1016/0002-8703(72)90445-0

[58] Grossman W, Jones D, McLaurin LP. Wall stress and patterns of hypertrophy in the human left ventricle. The Journal of Clinical Investigation. 1975;**56**(1):56-64. DOI: 10.1172/JCI108079

[59] Chung EE, Dianzumba SB, Morais P, Serjeant GR. Cardiac performance in children with homozygous sickle cell disease. Journal of the American College of Cardiology. 1987;**9**(5):1038-1042. DOI: 10.1016/s0735-1097(87)80305-4

[60] Caldas MC, Meira ZA, Barbosa MM. Evaluation of 107 patients with sickle cell anemia through tissue Doppler and myocardial performance index. Journal of the American Society of Echocardiography: Official Publication of the American Society of Echocardiography. 2008;**21**(10):1163-1167. DOI: 10.1016/j.echo.2007.06.001

[61] Sachdev V, Rosing DR, Thein SL. Cardiovascular complications of sickle cell disease. Trends in Cardiovascular Medicine. 2021;**31**(3):187-193. DOI: 10.1016/j.tcm.2020.02.002

[62] Lamers L, Ensing G, Pignatelli R, Goldberg C, Bezold L, Ayres N, et al. Evaluation of left ventricular systolic function in pediatric sickle cell anemia patients using the end-systolic wall stress-velocity of circumferential fiber shortening relationship. Journal of the American College of Cardiology. 2006;**47**(11):2283-2288. DOI: 10.1016/j.jacc.2006.03.005

[63] Di Maria MV, Hsu HH, Al-Naami G, Gruenwald J, Kirby KS, Kirkham FJ, et al. Left ventricular rotational mechanics in Tanzanian children with sickle cell disease. Journal of the American Society of Echocardiography. 2015;**28**(3):340-346. DOI: 10.1016/j.echo.2014.11.014

[64] Braga JC, Assef JE, Waib PH, de Sousa AG, de Mattos Barretto RB, Guimarães Filho FV, et al. Altered left ventricular twist is associated with clinical severity in adults and adolescents with homozygous sickle cell anemia. Journal of the American Society of Echocardiography. 2015;**28**(6):692-699. DOI: 10.1016/j.echo.2015.01.019

[65] Anthi A, Machado RF, Jison ML, Taveira-Dasilva AM, Rubin LJ,

Hunter L, et al. Hemodynamic and functional assessment of patients with sickle cell disease and pulmonary hypertension. American Journal of Respiratory and Critical Care Medicine. 2007;**175**(12):1272-1279. DOI: 10.1164/rccm.200610-1498OC

[66] Castro O, Hoque M, Brown BD. Pulmonary hypertension in sickle cell disease: Cardiac catheterization results and survival. Blood. 2003;**101**(4):1257-1261. DOI: 10.1182/blood-2002-03-0948

[67] Zilberman MV, Du W, Das S, Sarnaik SA. Evaluation of left ventricular diastolic function in pediatric sickle cell disease patients. American Journal of Hematology. 2007;**82**(6):433-438. DOI: 10.1002/ajh.20866

[68] Olson M, Hebson C, Ehrlich A, New T, Sachdeva R. Tissue Doppler imaging-derived diastolic function assessment in children with sickle cell disease and its relationship with ferritin. Journal of Pediatric Hematology/Oncology. 2016;**38**(1):17-21. DOI: 10.1097/MPH.0000000000000430

[69] Alsaied T, Niss O, Tretter JT, Powell AW, Chin C, Fleck RJ, et al. Left atrial dysfunction in sickle cell anemia is associated with diffuse myocardial fibrosis, increased right ventricular pressure and reduced exercise capacity. Scientific Reports. 2020;**10**(1):1767. DOI: 10.1038/s41598-020-58662-8. [Erratum in: Sci Rep. 2020 Mar 12;10(1):4880]

[70] Hankins JS, McCarville MB, Hillenbrand CM, Loeffler RB, Ware RE, Song R, et al. Ventricular diastolic dysfunction in sickle cell anemia is common but not associated with myocardial iron deposition. Pediatric Blood & Cancer. 2010;**55**(3):495-500. DOI: 10.1002/pbc.22587

[71] Johnson MC, Kirkham FJ, Redline S, Rosen CL, Yan Y, Roberts I, et al. Left ventricular hypertrophy and diastolic dysfunction in children with sickle cell disease are related to asleep and waking oxygen desaturation. Blood. 2010;**116**(1):16-21. DOI: 10.1182/blood-2009-06-227447

[72] Jhaveri S, Choueiter N, Manwani D, Ranabothu S, Morrone K, Hafeman M, et al. Association of anemia and blood pressure with novel markers of diastolic function in pediatric sickle cell disease. Journal of Pediatric Hematology/Oncology. 2021;**43**(4):e486-e493. DOI: 10.1097/MPH.0000000000002104

[73] Desai AA, Patel AR, Ahmad H, Groth JV, Thiruvoipati T, Turner K, et al. Mechanistic insights and characterization of sickle cell disease-associated cardiomyopathy. Circulation. Cardiovascular Imaging. 2014;**7**(3):430-437. DOI: 10.1161/CIRCIMAGING.113.001420

[74] Niss O, Fleck R, Makue F, Alsaied T, Desai P, Towbin JA, et al. Association between diffuse myocardial fibrosis and diastolic dysfunction in sickle cell anemia. Blood. 2017;**130**(2):205-213. DOI: 10.1182/blood-2017-02-767624

[75] Hayes MM, Vedamurthy A, George G, Dweik R, Klings ES, Machado RF, et al. American Thoracic Society implementation task force. Pulmonary hypertension in sickle cell disease. Annals of the American Thoracic Society. 2014;**11**(9):1488-1489. DOI: 10.1513/AnnalsATS.201408-405CME

[76] Gladwin MT, Barst RJ, Castro OL, Gordeuk VR, Hillery CA, Kato GJ, et al. Pulmonary hypertension and NO in sickle cell. Blood. 2010;**116**(5):852-854. DOI: 10.1182/blood-2010-04-282095

[77] Klings ES, Machado RF, Barst RJ, Morris CR, Mubarak KK, Gordeuk VR, et al. American Thoracic Society ad hoc committee on pulmonary hypertension of sickle cell disease. An official American Thoracic Society clinical practice guideline: Diagnosis, risk stratification, and management of pulmonary hypertension of sickle cell disease. American Journal of Respiratory and Critical Care Medicine. 2014;**189**(6):727-740. DOI: 10.1164/rccm.201401-0065ST

[78] Machado RF, Hildesheim M, Mendelsohn L, Remaley AT, Kato GJ, Gladwin MT. NT-pro brain natriuretic peptide levels and the risk of death in the cooperative study of sickle cell disease. British Journal of Haematology. 2011;**154**(4):512-520. DOI: 10.1111/j.1365-2141.2011.08777.x

[79] Takatsuki S, Ivy DD, Nuss R. Correlation of N-terminal fragment of B-type natriuretic peptide levels with clinical, laboratory, and echocardiographic abnormalities in children with sickle cell disease. The Journal of Pediatrics. 2012;**160**(3): 428-433.1. DOI: 10.1016/j.jpeds. 2011.09.015

[80] Machado RF, Anthi A, Steinberg MH, Bonds D, Sachdev V, Kato GJ, et al. N-terminal pro-brain natriuretic peptide levels and risk of death in sickle cell disease. Journal of the American Medical Association. 2006;**296**(3):310-318. DOI: 10.1001/jama.296.3.310

[81] Feld L, Fiorino EK, Aygun B, Appiah-Kubi A, Mitchell EC, Jackson S, et al. NT-proBNP levels and cardiopulmonary function in children with sickle cell disease. Pediatric Pulmonology. 2021;**56**(2):495-501. DOI: 10.1002/ppul.25155

[82] Onyekwere OC, Campbell A, Teshome M, Onyeagoro S, Sylvan C, Akintilo A, et al. Pulmonary hypertension in children and adolescents with sickle cell disease. Pediatric Cardiology. 2008;**29**(2):309-312. DOI: 10.1007/s00246-007-9018-x

[83] Zuckerman WA, Rosenzweig EB. Pulmonary hypertension in children with sickle cell disease. Expert Review of Respiratory Medicine. 2011;**5**(2):233-243. DOI: 10.1586/ers.11.6

[84] Yawn BP, Buchanan GR, Afenyi-Annan AN, Ballas SK, Hassell KL, James AH, et al. Management of sickle cell disease: Summary of the 2014 evidence-based report by expert panel members. JAMA. 2014;**312**(10):1033-1048. DOI: 10.1001/jama.2014.10517. Erratum in: JAMA. 2014 Nov 12;312(18):1932. Erratum in: JAMA. 2015 Feb 17;313(7):729

[85] Benza RL. Pulmonary hypertension associated with sickle cell disease: Pathophysiology and rationale for treatment. Lung. 2008;**186**(4):247-254. DOI: 10.1007/s00408-008-9092-8

[86] Rai P, Joshi VM, Goldberg JF, Yates AM, Okhomina VI, Penkert R, et al. Longitudinal effect of disease-modifying therapy on tricuspid regurgitant velocity in children with sickle cell anemia. Blood Advances. 2021;**5**(1):89-98. DOI: 10.1182/bloodadvances.2020003197

[87] Humbert M, Sitbon O, Simonneau G. Treatment of pulmonary arterial hypertension. The New England Journal of Medicine. 2004;**351**(14):1425-1436. DOI: 10.1056/NEJMra040291

[88] Barst RJ, Mubarak KK, Machado RF, Ataga KI, Benza RL, Castro O, et al. Exercise capacity and haemodynamics

in patients with sickle cell disease with pulmonary hypertension treated with bosentan: Results of the ASSET studies. British Journal of Haematology. 2010;**149**(3):426-435. DOI: 10.1111/j.1365-2141.2010.08097.x

[89] Machado RF, Barst RJ, Yovetich NA, Hassell KL, Kato GJ, Gordeuk VR, et al. Hospitalization for pain in patients with sickle cell disease treated with sildenafil for elevated TRV and low exercise capacity. Blood. 2011;**118**(4):855-864. DOI: 10.1182/blood-2010-09-306167

[90] Mehari A, Gladwin MT, Tian X, Machado RF, Kato GJ. Mortality in adults with sickle cell disease and pulmonary hypertension. Journal of the American Medical Association. 2012;**307**(12):1254-1256. DOI: 10.1001/jama.2012.358

[91] Gordeuk VR, Minniti CP, Nouraie M, Campbell AD, Rana SR, Luchtman-Jones L, et al. Elevated tricuspid regurgitation velocity and decline in exercise capacity over 22 months of follow up in children and adolescents with sickle cell anemia. Haematologica. 2011;**96**(1):33-40. DOI: 10.3324/haematol.2010.030767

[92] Ware RE, de Montalembert M, Tshilolo L, Abboud MR. Sickle cell disease. Lancet (London, England). 2017;**390**(10091):311-323. DOI: 10.1016/S0140-6736(17)30193-9

[93] Charache S, Terrin ML, Moore RD, Dover GJ, Barton FB, Eckert SV, et al. Effect of hydroxyurea on the frequency of painful crises in sickle cell anemia. Investigators of the multicenter study of hydroxyurea in sickle cell anemia. The New England Journal of Medicine. 1995;**332**(20):1317-1322. DOI: 10.1056/NEJM199505183322001

[94] Ware RE, Davis BR, Schultz WH, Brown RC, Aygun B, Sarnaik S, et al. Hydroxycarbamide versus chronic transfusion for maintenance of transcranial doppler flow velocities in children with sickle cell anaemia-TCD with transfusions changing to hydroxyurea (TWiTCH): A multicentre, open-label, phase 3, non-inferiority trial. Lancet. 2016;**387**(10019):661-670. DOI: 10.1016/S0140-6736(15)01041-7

[95] Wang WC, Ware RE, Miller ST, Iyer RV, Casella JF, Minniti CP, et al. Hydroxycarbamide in very young children with sickle-cell anaemia: A multicentre, randomised, controlled trial (BABY HUG). Lancet. 2011;**377**(9778):1663-1672. DOI: 10.1016/S0140-6736(11)60355-3

[96] Meier ER, Creary SE, Heeney MM, Dong M, Appiah-Kubi AO, Nelson SC, et al. Hydroxyurea optimization through precision study (HOPS): Study protocol for a randomized, multicenter trial in children with sickle cell anemia. Trials. 2020;**21**(1):983. DOI: 10.1186/s13063-020-04912-z

[97] Vichinsky E, Hoppe CC, Ataga KI, Ware RE, Nduba V, El-Beshlawy A, et al. A phase 3 randomized trial of voxelotor in sickle cell disease. The New England Journal of Medicine. 2019;**381**(6):509-519. DOI: 10.1056/NEJMoa1903212

[98] Henry ER, Metaferia B, Li Q, Harper J, Best RB, Glass KE, et al. Treatment of sickle cell disease by increasing oxygen affinity of hemoglobin. Blood. 2021;**138**(13):1172-1181. DOI: 10.1182/blood.2021012070

[99] Ataga KI, Kutlar A, Kanter J, Liles D, Cancado R, Friedrisch J, et al. Crizanlizumab for the prevention of pain crises in sickle cell disease. The New England Journal of Medicine. 2017;**376**(5):429-439. DOI: 10.1056/NEJMoa1611770. Epub 2016 Dec 3

[100] Eapen M, Brazauskas R, Walters MC, et al. Effect of donor type and conditioning regimen intensity on allogeneic transplantation outcomes in patients with sickle cell disease: A retrospective multicentre, cohort study. The Lancet. Haematology. 2019;**6**(11):e585-e596. DOI: 10.1016/S2352-3026(19)30154-1

[101] Kanter J, Walters MC, Krishnamurti L, et al. Biologic and clinical efficacy of LentiGlobin for sickle cell disease. The New England Journal of Medicine. 2022;**386**(7):617-628. DOI: 10.1056/NEJMoa2117175

[102] Frangoul H, Altshuler D, Cappellini MD, Chen YS, Domm J, Eustace BK, et al. CRISPR-Cas9 gene editing for sickle cell disease and β-thalassemia. The New England Journal of Medicine. 2021;**384**(3):252-260. DOI: 10.1056/NEJMoa2031054

Chapter 4

Innovations in Sickle Cell Care: Navigating the Dynamic Treatment Landscape

Oluwafemi Ajoyemi Ala

Abstract

Sickle cell anemia (SCA) is a genetic blood disorder characterized by the presence of abnormal hemoglobin, leading to the formation of sickle-shaped red blood cells. This causes vaso-occlusive crises, chronic anemia, and organ damage. Recent advancements in SCA treatment, including genetic therapies like CRISPR-Cas9, stem cell transplantation, disease-modifying drugs such as hydroxyurea, and telemedicine, offer hope for improved patient outcomes. However, challenges such as access to care and high treatment costs persist. This review discusses recent advances in SCA treatment, highlighting the potential of these therapies to transform patient care and improve quality of life. SCA is a hereditary blood disorder caused by a mutation in the gene that encodes hemoglobin, a protein responsible for carrying oxygen in red blood cells. This leads to production of abnormal hemoglobin, hemoglobin S (HbS). When oxygen levels are low, HbS molecules can polymerize and cause red blood cells to become rigid and assume a sickle shape. These sickle-shaped cells can block blood flow, leading to vaso-occlusive crises, chronic anemia, and organ damage. Recent advancements in the treatment of sickle cell anemia have offered new hope for patients. However, on-going research activities offer hope for continued improvements in the management of this complex disease.

Keywords: sickle cell anemia, genetic therapies, hematopoietic stem cell, transplantation, disease-modifying drugs, telemedicine, sickle cell disease, gene

1. Introduction

Sickle cell anemia (SCA) is a hereditary blood disorder characterized by the presence of abnormal hemoglobin, which causes red blood cells to become rigid and assume a sickle shape. This leads to various complications, such as pain, organ damage, and increased risk of infections. SCA is caused by a mutation in the gene that encodes the beta-globin subunit of hemoglobin, resulting in the production of abnormal hemoglobin known as hemoglobin S (HbS) [1–3]. When oxygen levels are low, HbS molecules can polymerize and cause red blood cells to become stiff and sickle-shaped. These sickle cells are prone to breaking down prematurely, leading to anemia, and can also block blood flow, causing vaso-occlusive crises.

Historically, SCA was associated with high mortality rates, particularly in childhood [4, 5]. However, advances in the understanding of the disease and its management have led to significant improvements in outcomes for patients. The discovery of the genetic basis of SCA in the 1950s paved the way for the development of new treatment strategies. The introduction of penicillin prophylaxis in the 1980s significantly reduced the risk of infections, a major cause of morbidity and mortality in SCA patients.

In recent years, there has been a growing recognition of the need for comprehensive care for SCA patients, including preventive measures, early intervention, and on-going monitoring. This approach, known as comprehensive care, aims to prevent complications, manage symptoms, and improve the overall quality of life for SCA patients. Comprehensive care includes regular monitoring of growth and development, screening for complications such as stroke and kidney disease, and providing access to multidisciplinary care teams.

Advances in the management of SCA have also been driven by improvements in supportive care, such as blood transfusions, pain management, and management of acute chest syndrome, a serious complication of SCA characterized by inflammation and blockage of blood vessels in the lungs. The development of disease-modifying therapies, such as hydroxyurea, has also significantly improved outcomes for SCA patients by reducing the frequency of vaso-occlusive crises and the need for hospitalization.

Despite these advancements, challenges remain in the management of SCA. Access to care, particularly for patients in low-resource settings, remains a major barrier to optimal treatment. Additionally, the high cost of treatment can be prohibitive for many patients, particularly in countries without universal healthcare coverage. Furthermore, there is a need for more targeted therapies that address the underlying genetic and molecular mechanisms of SCA, as current treatments mainly focus on symptom management.

Thus, significant advancements have been made in the management of sickle cell anemia, leading to improved outcomes and quality of life for patients. However, there is still much work to be done to address the remaining challenges and develop more effective therapies for this complex and debilitating disease. Continued research, advocacy, and investment in healthcare infrastructure are crucial to improving care and outcomes for SCA patients worldwide.

2. Genetic therapies

Genetic therapies have emerged as a promising avenue for the treatment of sickle cell anemia (SCA). These therapies aim to address the underlying genetic mutation responsible for the disease, offering the potential for a cure or long-term management of symptoms. Recent advancements in genetic engineering techniques, such as CRISPR-Cas9, have sparked significant interest in the field of SCA treatment (**Table 1**) [7].

CRISPR-Cas9 is a revolutionary gene editing tool that allows for precise modification of the DNA sequence. In the context of SCA, CRISPR-Cas9 can be used to target and correct the specific mutation in the beta-globin gene that leads to the production of abnormal hemoglobin. Early studies using CRISPR-Cas9 in animal models of SCA have shown promising results, with a significant reduction in sickle cell-related complications (**Figure 1**).

Therapy	Description	Current Status
CRISPR-Cas9	Gene editing tool that allows for precise modification of the DNA sequence. Can be used to target and correct the specific mutation in the beta-globin gene in SCA patients.	Early stages of clinical trials; promising results so far
Gene Therapy	Uses lentiviral vectors to introduce a functional copy of the hemoglobin gene into hematopoietic stem cells. These modified stem cells can produce normal hemoglobin.	Early stages of development; promising results in trials

Table 1.
Overview of genetic therapies for sickle cell anemia [6].

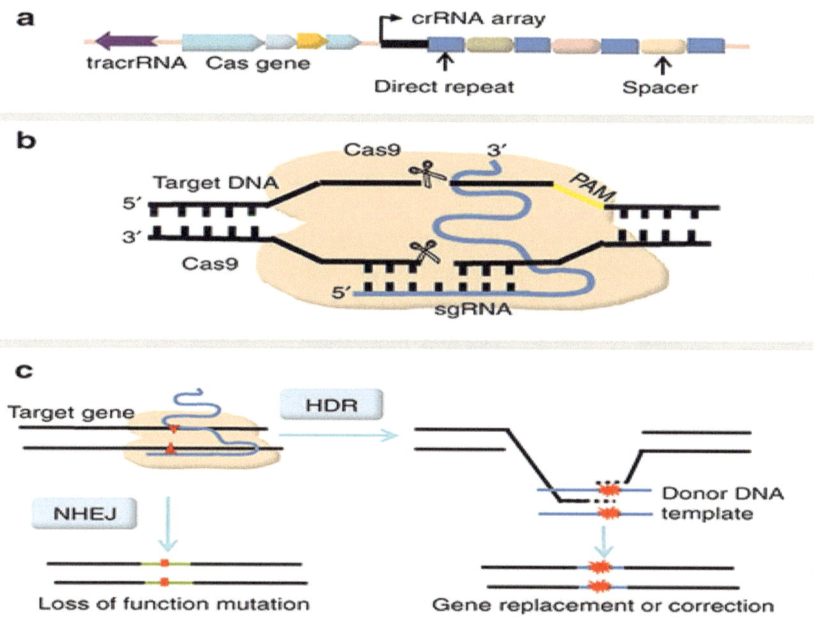

Figure 1.
Schematic Representation of CRISPR-Cas9 Gene Editing in Sickle Cell Anemia [6, 7]. [CRISPR-Cas9 Gene Editing in Sickle Cell Anemia] (https://example.com/crispr-cas9.jpg).

Early trials of gene therapy for SCA have shown promising results, with some patients achieving a significant reduction in sickle cell-related complications. However, like CRISPR-Cas9 therapy, gene therapy is still in the early stages of development, and more research is needed to determine its long-term safety and efficacy.

Figure 2 illustrates the process of CRISPR-Cas9 gene editing in sickle cell anemia. The CRISPR-Cas9 complex targets the specific mutation in the beta-globin gene, leading to a correction of the genetic defect and the production of normal hemoglobin.

Clinical trials using CRISPR-Cas9 in human patients with SCA are still in the early stages, but the results so far are encouraging. Some patients have experienced a complete remission of symptoms, including a reduction in the frequency of vaso-occlusive crises and an improvement in overall quality of life. However, more research is needed to fully understand the long-term effects and safety profile of CRISPR-Cas9 therapy in SCA patients.

In addition to CRISPR-Cas9, other genetic approaches are also being explored for the treatment of SCA. One such approach is gene therapy using lentiviral vectors to

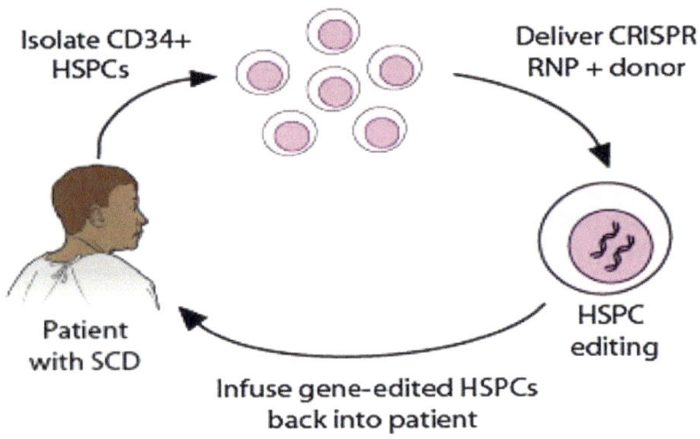

Figure 2.
Pictorial Analysis of Gene Editing in Sickle Cell Anemia Disease [7, 8].

introduce a functional copy of the hemoglobin gene into hematopoietic stem cells [7, 9]. These modified stem cells can then be transplanted back into the patient, where they can produce normal hemoglobin and replace the defective red blood cells.

Genetic therapies hold great promise for the treatment of sickle cell anemia. Advances in gene editing techniques such as CRISPR-Cas9 and gene therapy using lentiviral vectors offer new hope for patients with this debilitating disease [6]. While more research is needed to fully understand the long-term effects and safety of these therapies, the early results are promising, and genetic therapies may soon revolutionize the treatment of sickle cell anemia.

Thus, genetic therapies are at the forefront of sickle cell anemia treatment research, offering the potential for a cure or long-term management of symptoms. While still in the early stages of development, therapies such as CRISPR-Cas9 and gene therapy show promise in correcting the genetic defect underlying sickle cell anemia. Continued research and clinical trials are needed to fully understand the safety and efficacy of these therapies and to bring them to the patients who need them.

2.1 Stem cell transplantation

Hematopoietic stem cell transplantation (HSCT), also known as bone marrow transplantation, is a potentially curative treatment for sickle cell anemia (SCA), with the greatest cure rates attributed to this treatment plan. However, the use of HSCT is limited by the lack of suitable human leukocyte antigen (HLA)-matched donors and decreased application in older patients with significant morbidity (**Table 2**) [10, 11].

Myeloablative, HLA-identical sibling transplantation in children with sickle cell disease (SCD) offers excellent long-term survival, with overall and event-free survival rates of 95 and 92%, respectively. However, the risk of graft-versus-host-disease, infections, infertility, and other long-term transplant complications further limits its widespread use [12–14].

HSCT procedure involves replacing the patient's diseased bone marrow with healthy donor marrow that can produce normal hemoglobin. Stem cell transplantation offers the possibility of a permanent cure for SCA by providing a new source of healthy red blood cells.

Historically, stem cell transplantation was associated with significant risks, including graft rejection, graft-versus-host disease (GVHD), and transplant-related

Technique	Description	Advantages	Challenges
Reduced-intensity	Uses less toxic conditioning regimens, reducing the risk of complications such as graft rejection and GVHD.	Expanded pool of eligible donors, increased success rate of transplantation.	Limited availability in some regions, high cost of transplantation.
Gene-edited stem cells	Involves genetically modifying stem cells to correct the mutation that causes SCA.	Potential for a more precise and targeted treatment.	Limited availability, long-term effects unknown.
Haploidentical transplantation	Uses stem cells from a partially matched donor, typically a family member.	More readily available than fully matched donors.	Increased risk of GVHD, long-term effects unknown.

Table 2.
Comparison of stem cell transplantation techniques for sickle cell anemia [10, 11].

mortality. However, recent advancements in transplant techniques have significantly improved outcomes and reduced these risks. One such advancement is the use of reduced-intensity conditioning (RIC) regimens [15], which are less toxic than traditional conditioning regimens, allowing the extension of this modality to children and adults with significant morbidity [15–18]. This has expanded the pool of eligible donors and increased the success rate of transplantation. However, these approaches are also associated with an increased risk of graft failure. Thus, the optimal RIC regimen that strikes the optimal balance between maximizing the rate of stable engraftment while minimizing transplant-related morbidity and mortality is not fixed and thereby relatively unknown [5, 8, 16–21]. Alternative donor transplants, most prominently, partial HLA-mismatched related transplants (haploidentical), are being investigated with promising initial results [22].

In addition to reduced-intensity conditioning regimens, other advancements in stem cell transplantation for SCA include the use of gene-edited stem cells and haploidentical transplantation. Gene-edited stem cells are stem cells that have been genetically modified to correct the mutation that causes SCA. This approach offers the potential for a more precise and targeted treatment for SCA patients (**Figure 3**). Haploidentical transplantation involves using stem cells from a partially matched donor, typically a family member [5, 19–25]. This approach has the advantage of being more readily available than fully matched donors, making it a potentially more accessible treatment option for SCA patients.

Allogeneic transplant is curative for sickle cell anemia disease but has mainly been performed in children with severe disease, usually for overt strokes, recurrent acute chest syndrome, or recurrent vaso-occlusion pain episodes despite adherence to hydroxyurea therapy [21–27].

Also, for most of the cases seen globally, bone marrow-derived stem cells from HLA-matched sibling donors are primarily used, following myeloablative conditioning. Recent approaches are exploring the use of stem cells derived from blood, peripheral blood stem cells (PBSCT), and umbilical cord stem cells (UCBT) from a related newborn baby. Updates on the results of HLA-matched sibling HSCT for sickle cell disease performed worldwide between 1986 and 2013, reported to the European Blood and Marrow Transplant, Eurocord, and the Center for International Blood and Marrow Transplant Research (CIBMTR), were recently published [5, 8, 16–26]. More so, another benefit of HSCT includes abating progressive organ dysfunction [21–26], which is associated with early death in older patients with sickle cell anemia disease (**Table 3**).

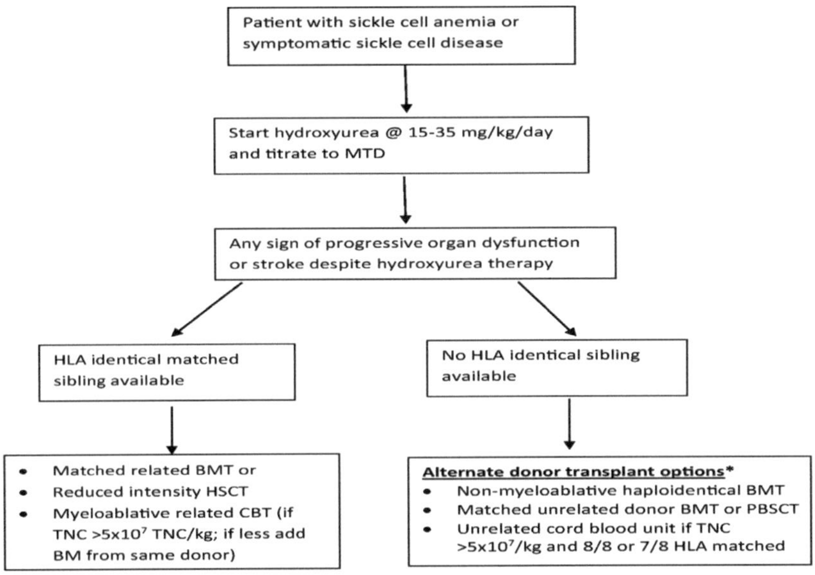

HSCT- hematopoietic stem cell transplant; BMT - bone marrow transplant; MTD - maximum tolerated dose; TNC – total nucleated cell count; CBT – cord blood transplant; BM – bone marrow PBSCT – peripheral blood stem cell transplant; HLA – human leukocyte antigen

* Choice of graft source and conditioning regimen may depend on institutional expertise; enrollment in clinical trials is strongly encouraged

Figure 3.
Suggested Approaches for HSCT for patients with Sickle Cell Anemia Disease [5, 8, 18–24].

It is worthy of note that for all genotypes, disease-related morbidity is the driving factor in pursuing an HSCT. Also, HSCT for adults with sickle cell disease is better tolerated with a low-intensity regimen but may require prolonged immune suppression to maintain stable mixed-donor chimerism (recipient and donor cells) (**Table 4**).

Clinical trials using these advanced stem cell transplantation techniques have shown promising results. Patients who have undergone stem cell transplantation have experienced a significant reduction in sickle cell-related complications and an improvement in overall quality of life. Some patients have even achieved a complete cure, with normal hemoglobin levels and no further need for transfusions.

Therefore, successful HSCT offers long-term protection from clinical and sub-clinical vaso-occlusion associated with sickle cell anemia disease, regardless of donor source, and minimizing late effects following HSCT is now a major therapeutic goal being constantly aimed. With a successful HSCT, end-organ complications that commonly develop in patients with sickle cell anemia disease, including stroke, pulmonary hypertension, acute chest syndrome, proteinuria, and haematuria, are usually not observed in patients after such transplant process, as defined by the stable engraftment of donor cells [23, 31–38].

Another major concern that has to be ruled out in order to measure the success of HSCT is gonadal insufficiency and infertility; specifically ovarian failure in females and low testosterone levels in males or hypogonadotropic hypogonadism. Thus, to ascertain the success of HSCT in this situation, health-related quality of life (QOL), which is determined by measures of physical, psychological, and social functioning, must have significantly improved after a certain period, starting from say 1 year, following successful HSCT.

Myeloablative matched sibling donor transplant and related cord blood transplant	Non-Myeloablative matched sibling donor transplant	Partially mismatched related donor (haploidentical) BMT
Advantages		
• Potential for cure • Large cumulative experience • Good rates of engraftment • Attenuates progressive • vasculopathy/end-organ damage • Disease-free survival: 85% • Overall survival: 97% • (Long follow up: 10–15 years)	• Does not exclude recipients with chronic organ damage • More applicable to adults with severe SCD • Disease-free survival: 79% • Overall survival: 95% • (Long follow up: 5–10 years)	• Does not exclude recipients with end-organ damage • Available to most patients (more than 50% of patients with SCD will have a suitable donor) • Disease-free survival: 58% • Overall survival: 100% • (Follow up: < 5 years)
Disadvantages		
• Limited availability (~10% of SCD patients with suitable donor) • Patient with end-organ damage usually excluded • Not recommended in adults with severe SCD • Graft rejection • Transplant-related mortality • Complications such as acute lung injury, infertility, endocrine and metabolic issues, and chronic GVHD	• Limited availability (~10% of SCD patients with suitable donor) • Higher risk of graft failure • Limited experience • Graft rejection • Transplant-related mortality • Late effects such as endocrine and metabolic issues and chronic GVHD	• Limited experience • Higher risk of graft rejection • Late effects

GVHD: Graft-versus-host disease; SCD: Sickle cell disease.

Table 3.
Advantages and disadvantages of different transplant approaches in patients with severe sickle cell disease [5, 12–14, 28, 29].

The successes recorded so far with HSCT concerning improved transplant outcomes for patients with sickle cell disease have also increased the demand for HSCT for patients with SCD from low-income countries, despite the huge cost implications. The HSCT demand is partly driven by the lack of standard care (hydroxyurea, chronic blood transfusion therapy, and comprehensive care programs) in their countries of origin, and is largely dependent on family preference and socio-economic status. However, facilities for both acute and late-effects management post-transplant are usually lacking in these low-income countries. Thus, following HSCT in high-income countries, patients living in low-income countries usually need long-term follow-up care abroad at significant costs. Medical facilities in low-income countries should address local challenges such as parasitaemia, malnutrition, availability of blood products, and other laboratory support services while developing a long-term strategy for managing patients who have undergone the procedure [33–37, 39, 40]. For patients residing in low-income countries seeking HSCT abroad, extensive discussion with the patient and family regarding the risk-benefit ratio, as well as a contingency plan to manage transplant-related complications for at least 2 years after the procedure at a hospital with adequate transplant expertise, are warranted.

Lastly in the section, there are still on-going trials that will help determine the true impact of HSCT on safety, progressive vasculopathy, and chronic organ dysfunction;

Matched sibling donor transplant	Matched unrelated donor transplant (MUD)	Partially mismatched related donor (haploidentical); unrelated cord blood transplant
Overt stroke or central nervous system event lasting >24 h	Overt stroke or any neurologic deficit lasting >24 h	Recurrent stroke despite adequate chronic blood transfusion therapy or progressive central nervous system changes
Impaired neuropsychological function with abnormal cerebral magnetic resonance imaging and angiography	Elevated TCD velocity unresponsive to hydroxyurea or chronic blood transfusion therapy	Severe SCD symptoms unresponsive to hydroxyurea therapy
Elevated TCD velocity unresponsive to hydroxyurea or chronic blood transfusion therapy	Recurrent acute chest syndrome despite hydroxyurea therapy	
Recurrent acute chest syndrome despite hydroxyurea therapy	Recurrent severe pain episodes despite hydroxyurea therapy	
Recurrent severe pain episodes despite hydroxyurea therapy	Red cell alloimmunization (transfusion support) plus established indication for chronic blood transfusion therapy	
Red cell alloimmunization plus established indication for chronic blood transfusion therapy	Pulmonary hypertension or an echocardiographic finding of tricuspid valve regurgitant jet velocity ≥ 2.7 m/s	
Pulmonary hypertension or an echocardiographic finding of tricuspid valve regurgitant jet velocity ≥ 2.7 m/s	Bone and joint involvement	
Recurrent priapism	Recurrent priapism	
Sickle nephropathy	Sickle nephropathy	
Bone and joint involvement		
Sickle retinopathy		
Stage I or II sickle cell lung disease		

AVN = avascular necrosis; TCD = transcranial Doppler; VOE = vaso-occlusive pain episodes; SCD: Sickle cell disease.

Table 4.
Current indications for HSCT in patients with severe sickle cell disease unresponsive to hydroxyurea therapy [22, 26, 30].

these will also help put more clarity and equally clear doubts as to whether patients with sickle cell anemia disease are at greater risk for declining organ function or whether RIC regimens offer better outcomes following HSCT. Thus, more research is needed to further improve the safety and efficacy of stem cell transplantation and to make it a more accessible treatment option for all sickle cell anemia patients.

3. Disease-modifying therapies

Disease-modifying therapies play a crucial role in the management of sickle cell anemia (SCA), aiming to reduce the frequency and severity of painful crises, improve quality of life, and prevent long-term complications. These therapies target various aspects of the underlying pathophysiology of SCA, including the production of abnormal hemoglobin and the adhesion of sickle cells to blood vessel walls, which worsen vaso-occlusion (**Table 5**) [23, 26, 31–37, 39, 42].

Hydroxyurea is one of the oldest and most widely used disease-modifying therapies for SCA. It works by increasing the production of foetal hemoglobin, which can substitute for the abnormal hemoglobin S and reduce sickle cell-related complications. Clinical studies have shown that hydroxyurea can reduce the frequency of painful crises, hospitalizations, and the need for blood transfusions in SCA patients. It is also associated with improvements in overall survival and quality of life.

Newer drugs, such as voxelotor (formerly known as GBT440) and crizanlizumab, offer more targeted approaches to treating SCA. Voxelotor is a hemoglobin oxygen affinity modulator that works by increasing the affinity of hemoglobin for oxygen, preventing the polymerization of hemoglobin S and the formation of sickle cells. Clinical trials have shown that voxelotor can significantly reduce the percentage of sickle cells in the blood and improve hemoglobin levels in SCA patients.

Crizanlizumab is a monoclonal antibody that targets P-selectin, a cell adhesion molecule involved in the adhesion of sickle cells to blood vessel walls. By inhibiting P-selectin, crizanlizumab reduces the adhesion of sickle cells and the formation of vaso-occlusive events. Clinical trials have demonstrated that crizanlizumab can reduce the frequency of painful crises and the need for hospitalizations in SCA patients [23, 26, 31–37, 39].

In addition to these pharmacological therapies, on-going research is exploring the use of gene therapy to boost the production of foetal hemoglobin and prevent sickle cell complications. Gene therapy approaches aim to introduce a functional copy of the hemoglobin gene into stem cells, allowing them to produce normal hemoglobin and reduce the production of abnormal hemoglobin S. Early studies using gene therapy for SCA have shown promising results, with some patients achieving sustained increases in foetal hemoglobin levels and improvements in clinical outcomes.

Table 6 illustrates the mechanism of action of disease-modifying therapies in sickle cell anemia. Hydroxyurea increases the production of foetal hemoglobin; voxelotor increases the affinity of hemoglobin for oxygen, and crizanlizumab targets P-selectin to reduce the adhesion of sickle cells to blood vessel walls.

Before concluding this section, it would be unfair not to mention the impact of pain initiatives and management in the assessment of sickle cell anemia disease. It is, therefore, imperative to understand the synergy of the drugs and therapies used in the management of pain with the other disease-modifying therapies; this synergy helps to get the best clinical, socio-economic, and humanistic outcomes from the management of sickle cell disease, and also equally promote the lives of the patients while seeking permanent answers in terms of therapies. Here below are some of the

Therapy	Mechanism of Action	Clinical Status
Hydroxyurea	Increases production of foetal hemoglobin, which can substitute for abnormal hemoglobin S.	Widely used; proven efficacy in clinical trials
Voxelotor	Increases the affinity of hemoglobin for oxygen, preventing the polymerization of hemoglobin S.	FDA-approved for the treatment of SCA
Crizanlizumab	Targets P-selectin, a cell adhesion molecule involved in the adhesion of sickle cells to blood vessel walls.	FDA-approved for the prevention of vaso-occlusive crises in SCA

Table 5.
Overview of few disease-modifying therapies for sickle cell anemia [26, 37, 41].

Medication	Mechanism of Action	Early Stages	Phase 2	Phase 3	Standard of care
Hydroxyurea	Targeting Hb S polymerization: increasing Hb F	→	→	→	→
*L-Glutamine (Endari) – FDA approved July 2017	Targeting vasoocclusion: Increase NAD and NADH and decrease adhesion	→	→	→	→
**Crizanlizumab (Adakveo) – FDA approved November 2019	Targeting vasoocclusion: P-selectin inhibition	→	→	→	→
**Voxelotor/ GBT440 (Oxbryta) – FDA approved November 2019	Targeting Hb S polymerization: increasing oxygen affinity	→	→	→	→
HLA-matched transplant	Modify the genotype	→	→	→	→
Haploidentical transplant	Modify the genotype	→	→	→	
***Rivipansel	Targeting vasoocclusion: Pan-selectin inhibition	→	→	→	
Sevuparin	Targeting vasoocclusion: Pan-selectin inhibition	→	→		
N-Acetylcisteine	Targeting inflammation: Antioxidant effect	→	→		
IMR-687	Targeting Hb S polymerization: inhibiting PDE9	→	→		
Sanguinate	Targeting Hb S polymerization: carbon monoxide delivery	→	→		
CRISPR-Cas9 modified CD34+	Modify the genotype	→			
Gamma-globin gene transfer	Modify the genotype	→			
Lentiglobin bb305	Modify the genotype	→			
Lentivirus shRNA targeting BCL11a	Modify the genotype	→			

** means FDA approved July 2017.*
*** means FDA approved November 2019.*
**** means Terminated in February 20, 2020 due to failure to meet primary endpoints.*

Table 6.
Mechanism of action of various disease-modifying therapies in sickle cell anemia [26, 43, 44].

illustrations of the efforts that have been made to standardize the management of pain globally and also discuss the processes involved in the management of severe pain, especially in an emergency room (**Figures 4** and **5**).

Therefore, disease-modifying therapies play a crucial role in the management of sickle cell anemia, offering targeted approaches to reduce the frequency and severity of complications. Hydroxyurea, voxelotor, and crizanlizumab, are examples of therapies that have shown promise in improving outcomes for SCA patients. On-going research into gene therapy holds the potential to further improve treatment options and ultimately find a cure for this complex and debilitating disease.

4. Telemedicine and remote monitoring

Telemedicine and remote monitoring have transformed the landscape of sickle cell anemia (SCA) management, offering new avenues for patient care, particularly in rural and underserved areas. These technologies encompass a wide range of

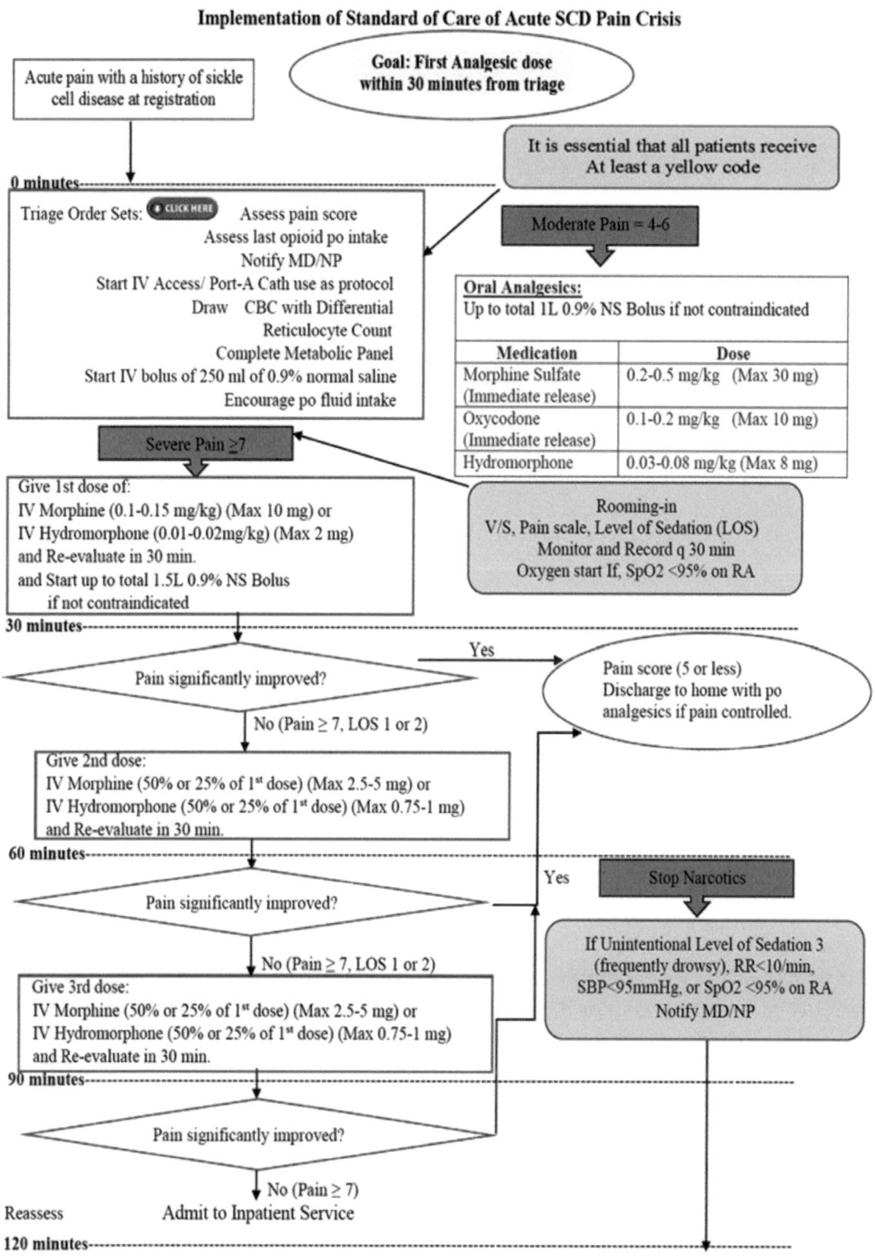

Figure 4.
Evidenced-Based Standard Practice of Care Algorithm for Vaso-Occlusive Pain Episodes [26, 45–47].

applications, including virtual consultations, remote monitoring of vital signs, and electronic health record (EHR) systems, all of which contribute to improved patient outcomes and quality of life.

One of the key advantages of telemedicine in SCA management is its ability to bridge the gap between patients and healthcare providers, allowing for more frequent and convenient access to care. This is especially important for SCA patients, who often require regular monitoring and may experience sudden severe symptoms that

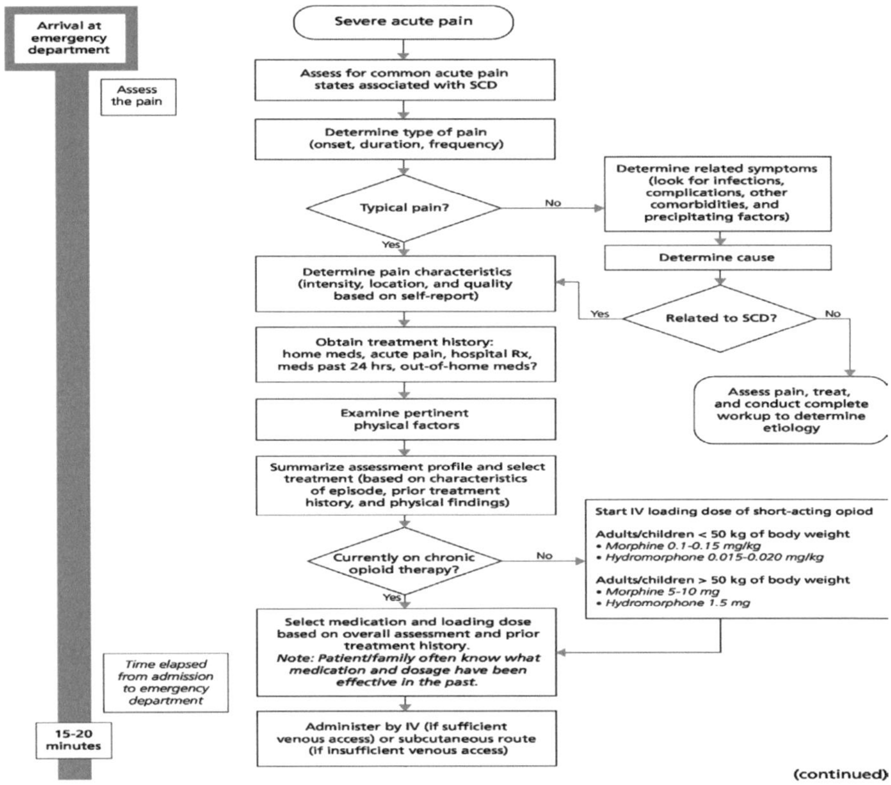

Figure 5.
Chart of Severe Acute Pain Management for Sickle Cell Disease in the Emergency Room [45, 46, 48, 49].

necessitate immediate attention. Telemedicine enables patients to consult with healthcare providers remotely, reducing the need for frequent hospital visits and improving overall adherence to treatment regimens.

Remote monitoring technologies also play a crucial role in SCA management, allowing for the continuous monitoring of vital signs and disease progression. For example, wearable devices can track parameters such as heart rate, oxygen saturation, and activity levels, providing valuable insights into a patient's health status. These devices can alert healthcare providers to potential complications, enabling early intervention and preventing serious health issues.

In addition to improving patient care, telemedicine and remote monitoring technologies have facilitated the participation of SCA patients in clinical trials and research studies (**Table 7**). By allowing patients to participate remotely, these technologies have expanded the pool of eligible participants and increased the diversity of study populations, leading to a better understanding of the disease and its treatment.

With the use of telemedicine and remote monitoring technologies in the management of sickle cell anemia, patients can consult with healthcare providers, access medical records, and monitor their condition remotely, improving overall health outcomes and quality of life.

Looking ahead, future advancements in telemedicine hold the potential to further enhance patient care and support for those living with SCA. For example, artificial intelligence (AI) algorithms can analyze large datasets of patient information to identify patterns and predict disease progression, enabling more personalized treatment

Benefit	Description
Increased access to care	Allows patients in rural and underserved areas to consult with healthcare providers remotely.
Improved adherence to treatment	Enables patients to monitor their condition and adhere to treatment regimens more effectively.
Enhanced patient engagement	Encourages patients to take a more active role in managing their health and well-being.
Early detection of complications	Allows for the early detection of potential complications, enabling timely intervention.
Facilitates participation in clinical trials	Enables patients to participate in clinical trials and research studies remotely.

Table 7.
Benefits of telemedicine and remote monitoring in sickle cell anemia management [48, 50].

approaches. Additionally, telemedicine platforms can be integrated with EHR systems to provide a seamless and comprehensive view of a patient's health history, enabling more informed decision-making by healthcare providers.

Thus, telemedicine and remote monitoring technologies have revolutionized the management of sickle cell anemia, offering new opportunities for patient care and support. These technologies have improved access to care, adherence to treatment, and patient engagement, leading to better outcomes for SCA patients. Continued advancements in telemedicine hold the potential to further enhance patient care and support for those living with this complex and challenging disease.

5. Patient education and support programs

Patient education and support programs play a critical role in the management of sickle cell anemia (SCA), empowering patients to take control of their health and improve their quality of life. These programs provide a range of services, including disease education, lifestyle modification guidance, and psychosocial support, all aimed at helping patients cope with the challenges of living with a chronic illness.

One of the key components of patient education programs is disease management education. Patients with SCA often require specialized care to manage their condition effectively. Education programs provide patients with information about their disease, including its causes, symptoms, and treatment options. This information helps patients make informed decisions about their care and empowers them to communicate effectively with their healthcare providers.

Lifestyle modification guidance is another important aspect of patient education programs for SCA. Patients with SCA can benefit from making changes to their lifestyle, such as adopting a healthy diet, staying hydrated and avoiding activities that can trigger a sickle cell crisis. Education programs provide patients with practical tips and strategies for managing their lifestyle to minimize the impact of SCA on their daily lives.

Psychosocial support is also a crucial component of patient education programs for SCA. Living with a chronic illness can be challenging, and patients may experience feelings of isolation, anxiety, or depression. Education programs provide patients with the tools and resources they need to cope with these challenges, including access to mental health services, support groups, and counseling.

Patient engagement in their care is a key goal of patient education programs for SCA. Studies have shown that patients who are actively involved in their care are more likely to adhere to their treatment regimens and achieve better health outcomes. Patient education programs help patients develop the skills and confidence they need to actively participate in their care, leading to improved overall health and well-being.

Peer support networks and advocacy groups also play a vital role in supporting patients with SCA. These groups provide a platform for patients to connect with others who are living with the same condition, share experiences, and provide mutual support. Peer support networks and advocacy groups also work to raise awareness about SCA and advocate for better access to care and treatment for patients.

Table 8 illustrates the components of patient education and support programs for sickle cell anemia, including disease management education, lifestyle modification guidance, psychosocial support, and patient engagement.

It would be unfair to conclude this section without mentioning the influence of the attitude of patients, the level of knowledge of sickle cell anemia disease by health-care providers who are crucial stakeholders, and the overall social determinants of treatment-seeking traits among the disease sufferers, as they all impact on the health outcomes and education of patients in terms of symptoms prevention and/or alleviation, as well as the reduction in rates of incessant hospitalization.

Figures 6 and 7 are meant to further explain some issues surrounding the knowledge of health workers, attitude of patients, and some social determinants as highlighted.

Component	Description
Disease management education	Provides information about the causes, symptoms, and treatment options for sickle cell anemia.
Lifestyle modification guidance	Offers practical tips and strategies for managing lifestyle factors that can impact SCA.
Psychosocial support	Provides access to mental health services, support groups, and counseling for emotional support.
Patient engagement	Empowers patients to take an active role in their care and make informed decisions about treatment.

Table 8.
Components of patient education and support programs for sickle cell anemia [24, 31, 35, 51].

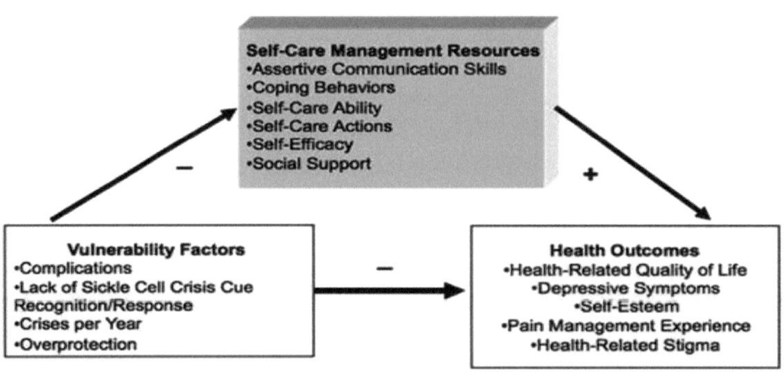

Figure 6.
Theory of Self-Care Management for Sickle Cell Disease [36, 39].

DOI: http://dx.doi.org/10.5772/intechopen.1005752

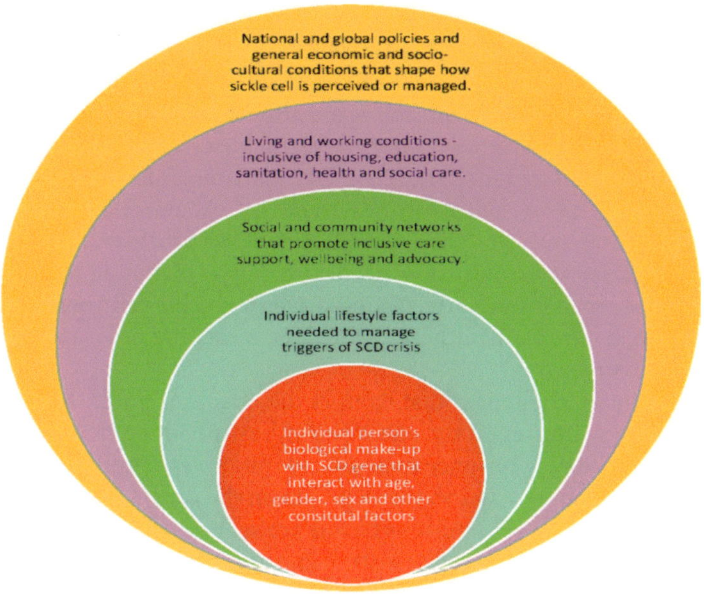

Figure 7.
Social Determinants of Sickle Cell Disorders – The Sickle Cell, Individual, Community Knowledge and Environment (SICKLE) Model [36, 39, 52].

Therefore, patient education and support programs are essential for empowering patients with sickle cell anemia, in order to manage their condition effectively. These programs provide patients with the information, tools, and support they need to cope with the challenges of living with a chronic illness. By educating and supporting patients, these programs help to improve treatment adherence, health outcomes, and overall quality of life for individuals with sickle cell anemia.

6. Public health initiatives

Public health initiatives are crucial in addressing the challenges of sickle cell anemia (SCA) by raising awareness, improving access to care, and supporting affected individuals and communities. These initiatives encompass a range of strategies, including education, screening, and advocacy, aimed at reducing the burden of SCA and improving outcomes for patients [23, 31–37, 39].

One of the key components of public health initiatives for SCA is raising awareness about the disease among healthcare providers, policymakers, and the general public. Many people are unaware of the impact of SCA and the importance of early diagnosis and treatment. Public health campaigns can help educate the public about SCA, its symptoms, and the available treatment options, leading to earlier diagnosis and better outcomes for patients.

Efforts to educate healthcare providers about SCA are also critical. Many healthcare providers may not be familiar with the unique challenges faced by patients with SCA or the latest treatment guidelines [36, 37]. Public health initiatives can provide training and resources to healthcare providers to improve their knowledge and understanding of SCA, leading to better care for patients.

Screening programs are another important component of public health initiatives for SCA. Screening can help identify individuals with SCA or sickle cell trait carriers, allowing for early intervention and treatment [36]. Screening programs can also provide valuable data for public health researchers to better understand the prevalence of SCA and its impact on communities [36–37, 39].

Family planning and genetic counseling are also key aspects of public health initiatives for SCA. Individuals who are carriers of the sickle cell trait have a 25% chance of passing the disease on to their children if their partner is also a carrier. Genetic counseling can help individuals understand their risk and make informed decisions about family planning, reducing the prevalence of SCA in future generations.

Such other information as seen above will also help to elaborate the importance of the various components of public health initiatives for sickle cell anemia, including raising awareness, educating healthcare providers, screening programs, family planning, and genetic counseling.

In likewise manner, challenges that hamper the effects of public health initiatives can also have a lasting impact on the outcomes of health, both either expected or unintended as the case may be, once policies and initiatives are distorted (**Table 9**).

Furthermore, assessment and analysis of data on the causes of death as well as the path to death of sickle cell disease sufferers are very important in public health research, as these will help to give futuristic projections to causes of mortalities and possible ways of avoiding such future occurrences (**Figure 8**) (**Table 10**).

Challenges/Burden of SCD in Nigeria	Government policies and programmes to address the challenges
• The 2018 National Demographic Health Survey (NDHS) report for the country put the prevalence of SCD to be highest in the South West (2%), lowest in the South (0.3%) and 21% HbAS and 5% HbAC for southwest and overall prevalence of 1% among the children below 5 years	• Establishment of six zonal Centres of Excellence for SCD which are equipped with HPLC for early detection and comprehensive care of diagnosed babies
	• Creation of a National Desk for SCD at the FMoH
	• Review of the existing National Guideline for the Management and Control of SCD
• SCD is among the top 10 non-communicable diseases (NCDs) causing significant disability, morbidity and mortality impacting negatively on the attainment of Sustainable Development Goals (SDGs) 1, 3, 4 and 10	• Protocol for the Universal Newborn Screening for SCD
• Poor integration of SCD prevention and control services with other health and nonhealth services especially maternal and child health services	• Expansion of the national immunization schedule to include pneumococcal and influenza vaccination for children with SCD
• Cultural beliefs and ignorance (myths) about SCD across the country	• Launching of the National Multisectoral Action Plan for SCD and other Prioritized NCDs
• Too many uncoordinated activities of NGOs in SCD community in Nigeria	• Streamlining and coordinating activities of NGO/CSOs in the SCD community
• Non-prioritization of SCD due to poor understanding of the contribution and linkage of the disease to poverty and mortality indices in Nigeria by the major development partners	• High level advocacy resulting in legislative frameworks that ensure SCD is accorded priority attention required considering the high burden of the disease
• Inability of government to mobilize the much-needed resources for SCD interventions	• Multilateral collaboration and partnerships with international organization such as WHO and local industries and NGOs
	• Scaling up high level advocacy and dialog for SCD

Table 9.
Example of feedback from policymakers (hospital management staff and government representatives from Nigeria's Federal Ministry of Health) to assess the challenges and resolutions [19, 35, 45].

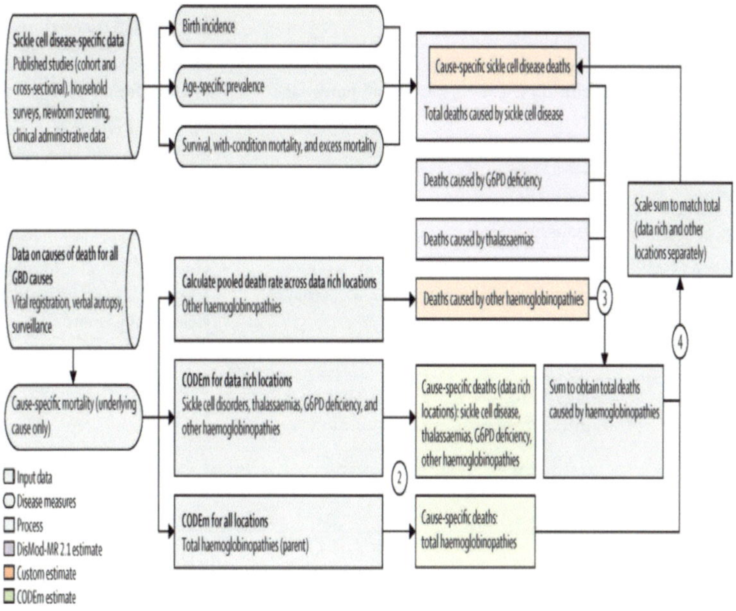

Figure 8.
Flowchart showing prevalence, cause-specific mortality, and total sickle cell disease mortality estimation process [35, 45, 48, 53].

Experience/Challenges	Strategies/Expectations
Access	• Provision of more specialized sickle cell centres • Capacity building, enhancement, and job protection for health workers to enable them put in their best
• Delay before accessing care. Quantified to be about 2 h or more before talking to a doctor. Turnaround time for investigations can take up to 3 days for one consultation • Difficulty in accessing a preferred healthcare worker	
• Healthcare workers are unfriendly	
• Specialist SCD centres are few and difficult to access • Unorthodox, and uncertified care is very much available and easy to access	
Contextual knowledge (knowledge of healthcare providers on needs of patients)	• Every clinic day should be a unique journey with exciting new things to look forward to
• Family support is poor • Clinic days are too routine and rigid and often difficult to fit into individual patient's schedules	
Communication	• Provision of more specialized sickle cell centres and employment of more healthcare providers especially social workers and haemoglobinopathy counselors
• Healthcare workers are too much in a hurry to write drugs and dismiss a patient without listening to the problems of the patient • The guinea pig mentality. Sometimes patients believe that everything done for the patient is just to make him/her give blood for research	
Comprehensiveness	
• Consultations not holistic as social and spiritual issues are seldom attended to	• Multidisciplinary team management

Experience/Challenges	Strategies/Expectations
• Lack of counseling that may lead to the philosophy "once I am fine, no need to go to the clinic", self-medication and patronage of quacks may then follow	• Health education and public enlightenment for all • Improvement of emergency care and blood transfusion services
• Stigma	
Coordination	
Emergency care and blood transfusion are inefficient	
• The National Health Insurance Service (NHIS) is unfriendly to patients. Many times, routine drugs for SCD are not available in the scheme or out of stock	• Government should make NHIS more friendly and effectively accommodate sickle cell patient
• **High cost of services**	• Increase health insurance coverage and inclusion of hydroxyurea in NHIS drugs list
• Cost implications, an average of 10,000 naira ($20) on drugs monthly, excluding transport, investigations, consultation fee and others	
• Important drugs for care such as hydroxyurea are expensive and difficult to access	

Table 10.
Quality of healthcare services (examples of feedback from patients' care givers, patients, and support non-governmental organizations in some hospitals in Nigeria) [19, 35, 45, 54].

Thus, public health initiatives play a critical role in addressing the challenges of sickle cell anemia by raising awareness, improving access to care, and supporting affected individuals and communities. Continued investment in these initiatives is essential to reduce the burden of SCA globally and improve outcomes for patients.

7. Collaborative research efforts

Collaborative research efforts have been instrumental in advancing our understanding of sickle cell anemia (SCA) and developing new treatment options for this complex disease. These collaborative efforts involve partnerships between academia, industry, and patient advocacy groups, bringing together diverse expertise and resources to address the challenges of SCA comprehensively.

One of the key outcomes of collaborative research efforts in SCA is the identification of novel drug targets. Researchers have identified specific pathways and molecules involved in the pathogenesis of SCA, leading to the development of targeted therapies that can modify the course of the disease. For example, drugs targeting the adhesion of sickle cells to blood vessel walls, such as crizanlizumab, have shown promise in reducing the frequency of vaso-occlusive crises in SCA patients (**Figures 9** and **10**).

List of some of the therapies and drugs developed through collaborative efforts is shown in **Table 11**.

Another important outcome of collaborative research efforts is the development of innovative therapies for SCA. Gene therapy, for example, offers the potential for a cure by introducing a functional copy of the hemoglobin gene into stem cells, allowing them to produce normal hemoglobin. Clinical trials using gene therapy for SCA have shown promising results, with some patients achieving sustained increases in foetal hemoglobin levels and improvements in clinical outcomes. Another beauty of world-class collaborative efforts that resulted in a major breakthrough is the gene therapy and editing process towards the erasing of sickle cell anemia disease.

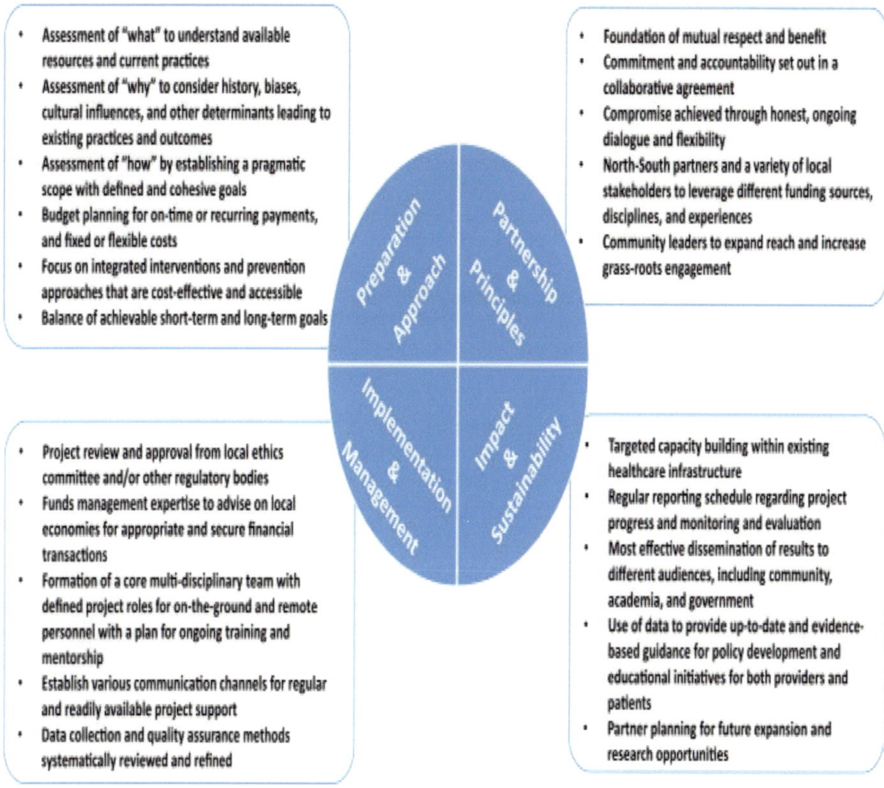

Figure 9.
Translating Clinical Care of Sickle Cell Disease to low-resource Countries through International Research Collaborations (A) [45, 48].

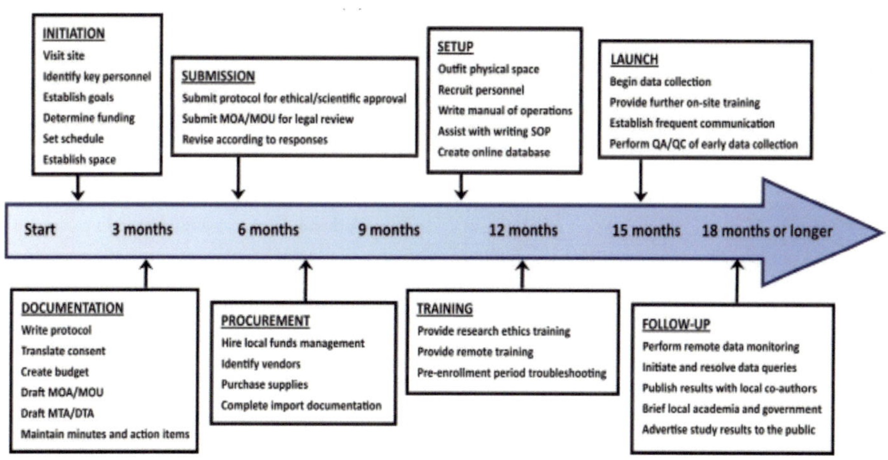

Figure 10.
Translating Clinical Care of Sickle Cell Disease to low-resource Countries through International Research Collaborations (B) [45, 48].

Figure 11 illustrates the collaborative nature of research efforts in sickle cell anemia, involving partnerships between academia, industry, and patient advocacy groups.

Drug compound	Drug action
Target: Erythrocyte rheology. Reducing polymerization, and improving cellular hydration	
Hydroxyurea*	Increases HbF. reduces HbS polymerization
Senicapoc*	Improves RBC dehydration
Metformin*	Increases HbF
Aes-103*	Prevents HbS polymerization
Voxelotor*	Prevents HbS polymerization
Target: Reducing cellular adhesion and vaso-occlusion	
Hydroxyurea*	Improves red cell rheology
Crizanlizumab*	P-selectin inhibitor
Rivipansel*	Pan-selectin inhibitor
Intravenous lg*	Neutrophil integrin Mac-1 inhibition
Tinzaparin*	Reduces RBC adhesion
Dalteparin*	Reduces RBC adhesion
Sevuparin*	Reduces RBC adhesion
Eptifibatide*	Inhibits platelet aggregation
NKTT120*	iNKT-blocking monoclonal antibody
Ticagrelor*	Inhibits platelet aggregation
Prasugrel*	Inhibits platelet aggregation
Target: improving endothelial dysfunction	
Hydroxyurea*	Nitric oxide donor
L-glutamine*	Nitric oxide donor
Haptoglobin*	Hemoglobin scavenger
Oral or intravenous nitrite*	Nitric oxide donor
Arginine*	Nitric oxide donor
Inhaled nitric oxide*	Nitric oxide donor
Antioxidants*	Reduce production of ROS
Target: Improving sterile inflammation	
Haemopexin/haptoglobin*	Haem/Hb-binding proteins, antioxidant
MP4CO*	Modulates HO-1 and inflammation
Various anti oxidants*	Reduce crisis and inflammation
TLR4-inhibition**	Mediates haem-induced inflammation
DNAse-1**	Dissolves NET produced by neutrophils
Canakinumab*	IL-1β inhibitor
Montelukast*	Cysteinyl leukotrienes receptor antagonist
Simvastatin*	Statin therapy to protect vascular endothelium
Anakinra**	IL-1 inhibitor

** means U.S. Food and Drug Administration (FDA).*
*** means Under investigation.*

Table 11.
Short list of currently approved drugs and study trials of potential future treatments for sickle cell disease through various collaborative efforts [26, 37, 55–57].

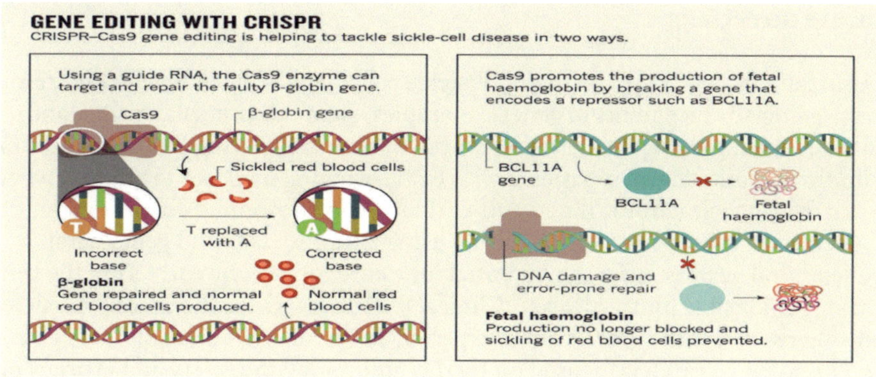

Figure 11.
Collaborative Efforts to Showcase the Beauty of Gene Therapy and Editing [58–63].

Large-scale clinical trials are also a key focus of collaborative research efforts in SCA. These trials are essential for evaluating the safety and efficacy of new treatments and providing evidence-based guidelines for clinical practice. Collaborative efforts between researchers, healthcare providers, and patient advocacy groups have enabled the initiation of large-scale clinical trials, such as the HOPE Study, which is evaluating the use of gene therapy in SCA patients.

On-going research is focused on developing curative therapies, improving transplant outcomes, and addressing the long-term complications of sickle cell disease.

Thus, collaborative research efforts have been instrumental in advancing our understanding of sickle cell anemia and developing new treatment options for this complex disease (**Figure 12**). By working together, researchers, healthcare providers, and patient advocacy groups are making significant strides towards improving the lives of individuals affected by sickle cell anemia.

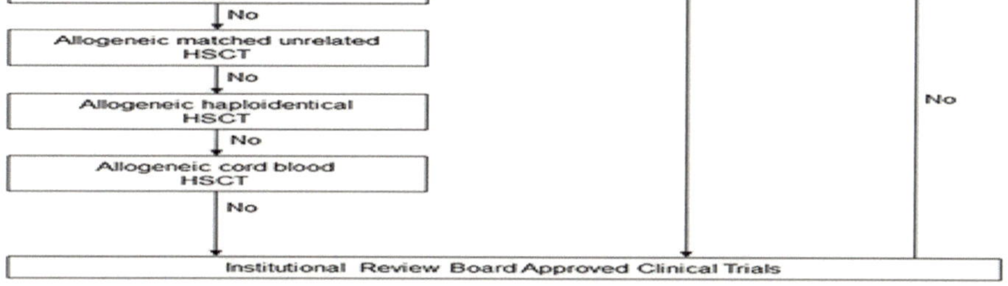
All patients with SCD
regardless of genotype and symptomatology
Curative Treatments
Non-Curative Treatments
Autologous HSCT with Gene Therapy
No
Allogeneic matched sibling HSCT
No
Allogeneic matched unrelated HSCT
No
Allogeneic haploidentical HSCT
No
Allogeneic cord blood HSCT
No
Symptomatic Therapies
Red Blood Cell Transfusions (Simple or Exchange)
Disease modifying drug therapies
No
Institutional Review Board Approved Clinical Trials

Figure 12.
Development of Curative Therapies for Sickle Cell Anemia Disease [22, 58–60].

8. Future directions

Future directions in the treatment of sickle cell anemia (SCA) hold great promise, with on-going advancements in genetic therapies, stem cell transplantation, and disease-modifying therapies. These advancements are expanding treatment options and improving outcomes for patients with SCA, bringing us closer to a future where SCA is a manageable chronic illness rather than a life-threatening condition.

Genetic therapies, such as gene editing using CRISPR-Cas9 and gene therapy using lentiviral vectors, offer the potential for a cure for SCA by correcting the genetic mutation responsible for the disease. Clinical trials using these therapies have shown promising results, with some patients experiencing a complete remission of symptoms. On-going research is focused on further improving the safety and efficacy of these therapies and expanding access to them for all SCA patients.

Stem cell transplantation remains the only cure for SCA, and recent advancements in transplant techniques, such as reduced-intensity conditioning regimens and haploidentical transplantation, have significantly improved outcomes and reduced risks associated with the procedure. On-going research is exploring new approaches to stem cell transplantation, such as the use of gene-edited stem cells, to further improve outcomes and expand access to transplantation for all SCA patients.

Disease-modifying therapies, such as hydroxyurea, voxelotor, and crizanlizumab, continue to be a cornerstone of SCA treatment, offering targeted approaches to reducing the frequency and severity of complications.

On-going research is focused on developing new disease-modifying therapies that target specific pathways involved in the pathogenesis of SCA, with the goal of further improving outcomes for patients.

Figure 13 illustrates the future directions in sickle cell anemia treatment, including advances in genetic therapies, stem cell transplantation, and disease-modifying therapies.

Advances in understanding the underlying mechanisms of SCA are also driving research towards more targeted and effective treatments. For example, researchers are investigating the role of oxidative stress, inflammation, and endothelial dysfunction in the pathophysiology of SCA, with the aim of developing new therapies that target these pathways. Additionally, research into the role of the microbiome in SCA may lead to new treatment strategies that modulate the gut microbiota to improve outcomes for patients.

The value of prevention in sickle cell anemia disease is important in several contexts. Pre-conception screening of couples to avoid high-risk pregnancies is recommended, and females need relevant information on how to manage their pregnancy for better outcomes. Studies have shown that the prevalence of ischaemic stroke by the age of 20 years is ≥11%, with the highest stroke rates occurring in early childhood. Transcranial Doppler ultrasound is also used to identify patients at the highest risk who may benefit from transfusion therapy [64, 65]. Prophylactic erythrocytapheresis addresses the problem of slow red blood cell transfusion, reducing the concentration of sickle hemoglobin-containing red cells, thereby improving symptoms of crises quickly [55]. For the prevention of infection in children with sickle cell anemia disease, prophylactic antibiotics initiated as early as 3 months of age are highly recommended.

Finally, the future of sickle cell anemia treatment holds great promise, with on-going advancements in genetic therapies, stem cell transplantation, and disease-modifying therapies. Continued investment in research and healthcare infrastructure is essential to realize this promise and ensure that all SCA patients have access to the

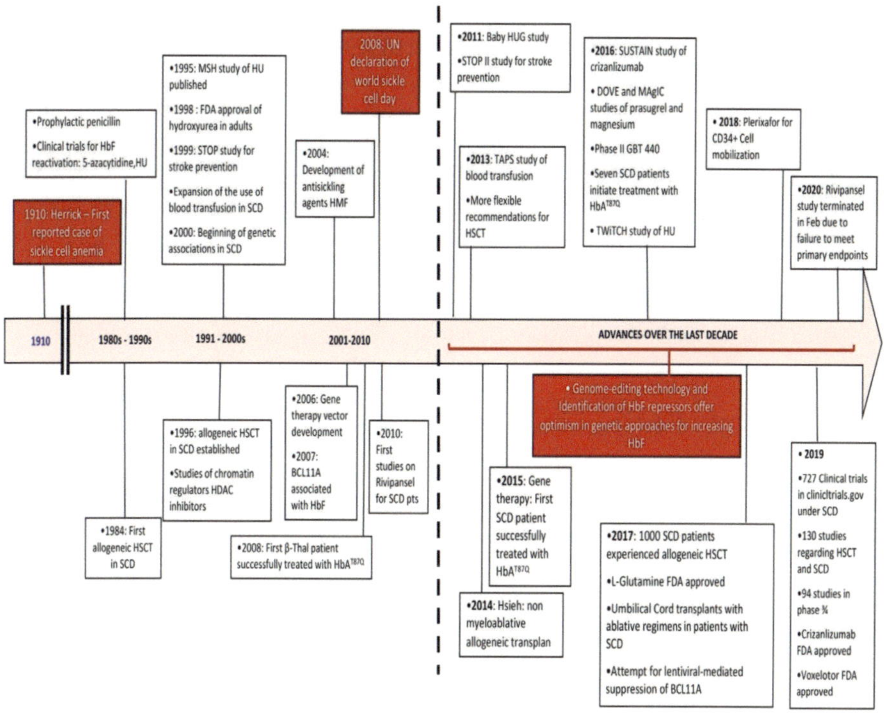

Figure 13.
Advances in Sickle Cell Anemia Disease over the last few Decades [22, 58–60].

latest and most effective treatments. Collaboration between researchers, healthcare providers, and patients is essential and also fundamentally key to achieving this goal and improving outcomes for individuals affected by SCA.

The field of sickle cell anemia healthcare and treatment has seen significant advancements in recent years, offering new hope for patients and improving their quality of life. However, sickle cell anemia disease is a global disease; it is no longer only a disease in developing countries but is becoming more widespread in Europe and across the world. For example, all through the period that the world experienced the devastating spread of SARS-CoV-2 (COVID-19), it was a major challenge for healthcare providers as the global pandemic presented unprecedented challenges in managing care for patients with sickle cell anemia disease. There are serious unmet needs to address if patients are to be treated successfully, especially because the pathophysiology of sickle cell anemia disease is extremely complex, making it difficult to find a unique treatment.

Also, there are a number of barriers to the management of vaso-occlusion and other associated challenges. Several studies showed that levels of patient pain are underestimated if they are only measured via healthcare facilities, indicating a need to improve patients' experiences of acute care. Studies have also shown that approximately, 25% of vaso-occlusion reported are most of the time managed by patients at home. From the patient's perspective, this is largely, but not exclusively, because of perceived poor medical experiences at the emergency room (ER) or hospital, which then prevent the patients from seeking further medical assistance when needed [48, 66].

In addition to the overcrowded and stressful hospital/ER environment, barriers to vaso-occlusion (VOC) management include poor transition from pediatric to adult care, the stigma associated with having sickle cell anemia disease, ethnicity, and requiring opioids for pain control. Patients with sickle cell anemia disease also wait longer to see an ER physician than, for example, a patient with a long bone fracture, which may be because of a lack of experience with sickle cell anemia disease, or a lack of empathy as a result of the aforementioned stigma (**Figure 14**).

Furthermore, the effects of medication on fertility rates and pregnancy are also of concern to patients. Most current research works have shown no clear evidence exists of a negative effect of hydroxyurea therapy on fertility, but further research is needed as more treated patients reach adulthood (**Figures 15** and **16**) [70, 71].

Optimum management of vaso-occlusion can be facilitated by pain action plans designed to educate patients on strategies to prevent triggers, advise on self-care

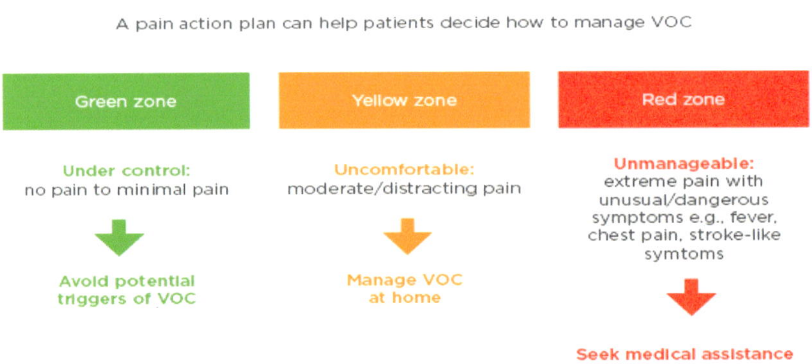

Figure 14.
Example of Pain Action Plan - Patients using Traffic Light Color Coding for Highlights [26, 45, 60, 67].

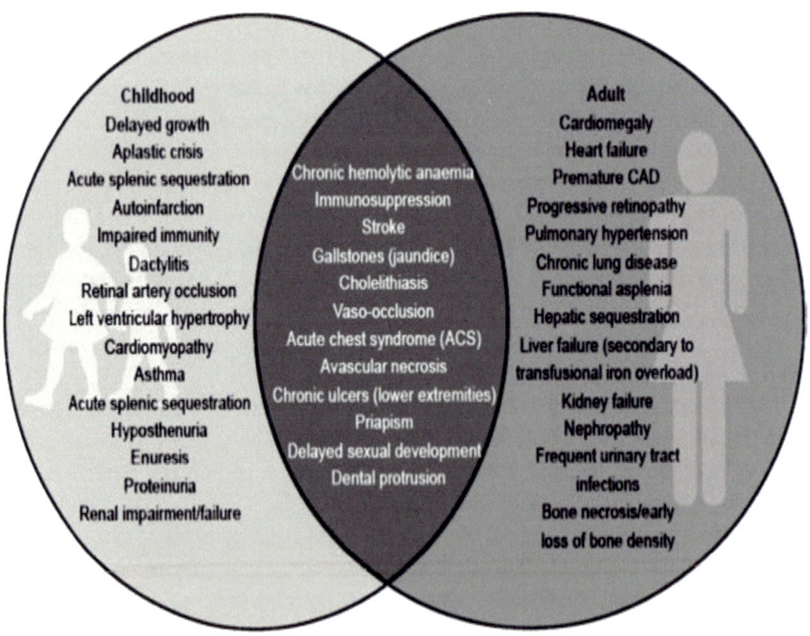

Figure 15.
Overview of Complications from Sickle Cell Disease – Childhood and Adulthood [22, 58–60, 68].

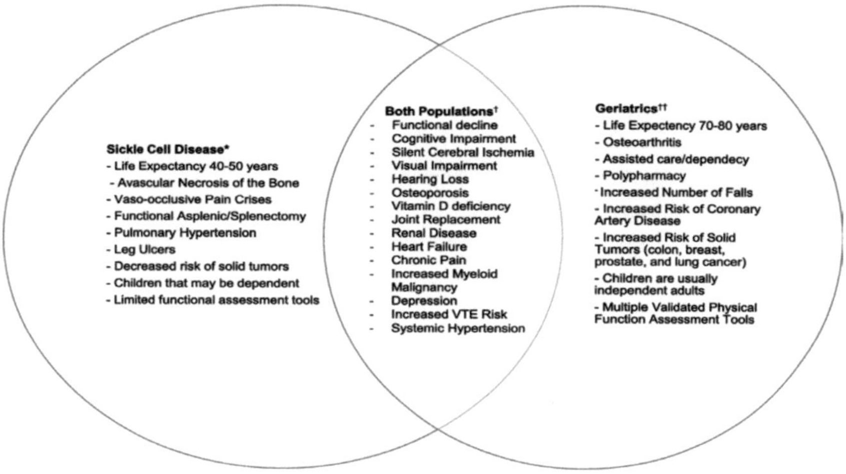

Figure 16.
Overview of the Comparison of the Characteristics and Complications of Sickle Cell Disease versus Geriatrics [22, 58–60, 69].

strategies to manage pain at home and inform patients when to seek medical assistance. Pain action plans also encompass guidance for acute pain management, discharge planning to prevent rebound-pain exacerbation, and co-ordination of care after discharge [45]. This preventative approach helps patients to recognize their pain severity and manage their vaso-occlusion accordingly (**Figure 17**).

Strategies to overcome these barriers include patient plans, day hospitals, and structured transition programmes. In this decade of new drug development, there is a need to examine the potential role of combination therapies. Hydroxyurea is a

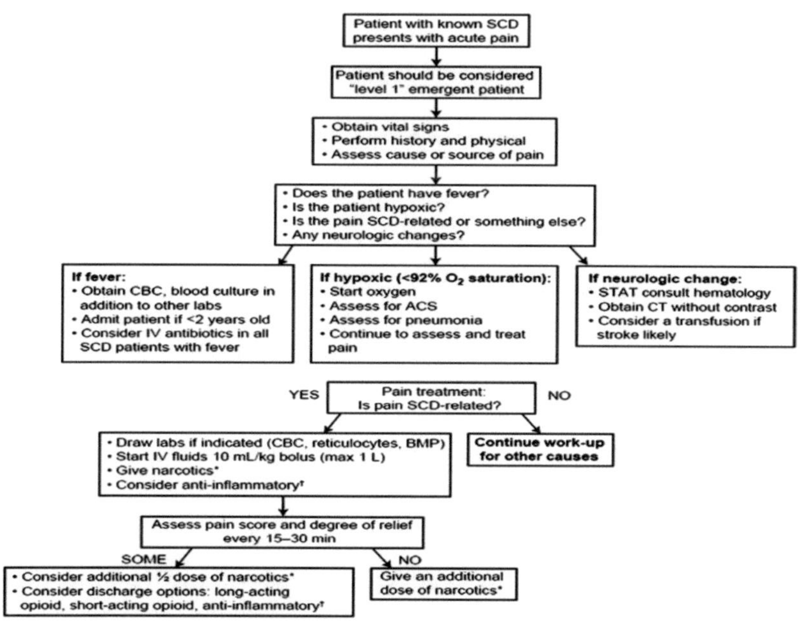

Figure 17.
Template - Clinical Management of Acute Pain and other aspects of Sickle Cell Disease [26, 45, 46, 60, 67].

well-established drug and most trials are based on patients already on this treatment; adding another drug may become the standard of care in the future [67, 72–75].

However, because of the global distribution of patients especially in developing countries, there is a need to consider the cost of new therapies. Many people do not have access to safe blood transfusions, therapeutic options, or even iron chelation and to address the unmet needs of sickle cell anemia disease worldwide, global collaboration is needed to develop treatments and protocols.

Thus, by working together, we can continue to advance the field and improve outcomes for individuals living with this challenging disease.

9. Summary of chapter/conclusion

Sickle cell anemia (SCA) is a complex genetic disorder that has historically posed significant challenges for patients and healthcare providers. However, recent advancements in SCA healthcare and treatment offer new hope for patients and are transforming the landscape of SCA management. This chapter has explored some of the key advancements in SCA treatment, including genetic therapies, stem cell transplantation, disease-modifying therapies, telemedicine, patient education and support programs, public health initiatives, collaborative research efforts, and future directions in SCA treatment.

Genetic therapies, such as gene editing using CRISPR-Cas9 and gene therapy using lentiviral vectors, offer the potential for a cure for SCA by correcting the genetic mutation responsible for the disease [58, 76]. These therapies have shown promising results in clinical trials, with some patients experiencing a complete remission of symptoms [59, 60].

Stem cell transplantation remains the only cure for SCA, and recent advancements in transplant techniques have significantly improved outcomes and reduced risks associated with the procedure [77–80].

Disease-modifying therapies, such as hydroxyurea, voxelotor [81, 82], and crizanlizumab, offer targeted approaches to reducing the frequency and severity of complications in SCA patients.

Telemedicine and remote monitoring technologies have revolutionized the management of SCA, especially in rural and underserved areas, by providing patients with access to healthcare providers, medical records, and condition monitoring remotely. Patient education and support programs have empowered patients with SCA to better manage their condition, providing information on disease management, lifestyle modifications, and psychosocial support [83, 84]. Public health initiatives aimed at raising awareness about SCA and improving access to care have played a crucial role in improving outcomes for patients, leading to earlier diagnosis and better treatment outcomes [85–88].

Collaborative research efforts between academia, industry, and patient advocacy groups have been instrumental in advancing our understanding of SCA and developing new treatment options. These partnerships have led to the identification of novel drug targets, the development of innovative therapies, and the initiation of large-scale clinical trials.

Future directions in SCA treatment hold great promise, with on-going advancements in genetic therapies, stem cell transplantation, and disease-modifying therapies.

DOI: http://dx.doi.org/10.5772/intechopen.1005752

Author details

Oluwafemi Ajoyemi Ala[1,2]

1 University College Hospital Ibadan, Nigeria

2 University of Ibadan, Nigeria

*Address all correspondence to: ala.oluwafemii@gmail.com;
oluwafemi.ala@uch-ibadan.org.ng

References

[1] Hassell KL. Population estimates of sickle cell disease in the US. American Journal of Preventive Medicine. 2010;**38**:S512-S521

[2] Eaton WA, Hofrichter J. Haemoglobin S gelation and sickle cell disease. Blood. 1987;**70**:1245-1266

[3] Platt OS, Thorington BD, Brambilla DJ, Milner PF, Rosse WF, Vichinsky E, et al. Pain in sickle cell disease. Rates and risk factors. The New England Journal of Medicine. 1991;**325**:11-16

[4] Platt OS, Brambilla DJ, Rosse WF, Milner PF, Castro O, Steinberg MH, et al. Mortality in sickle cell disease. Life expectancy and risk factors for early death. The New England Journal of Medicine. 1994;**330**:1639-1644

[5] Lanzkron S, Carroll CP, Haywood C. Mortality rates and age at death from sickle cell disease: U.S., 1979-2005. Public Health Reports. 2013;**128**:110-116

[6] Negre O, Eggimann AV, Beuzard Y, Ribeil JA, Bourget P, Borwornpinyo S, et al. Gene therapy of the beta-haemoglobinopathies by lentiviral transfer of the beta(A(T87Q))-globin gene. Human Gene Therapy. 2016;**27**:148-165. DOI: 10.1089/hum.2016.007

[7] Ribeil J, Hacein-Bey-Abina S, Payen E, Magnani A, Semeraro M, Magrin E, et al. Gene therapy in a patient with sickle cell disease. The New England Journal of Medicine. 2017;**376**:848-855

[8] Humbert O, Radtke S, Samuelson C, Carrillo RR, Perez AM, Reddy SS, et al. Therapeutically relevant engraftment of a CRISPR-Cas9–edited HSC-enriched population with HbF reactivation in nonhuman primates. Science Translational Medicine. 2019;**11**:eaaw3768

[9] CRISPR-Cas9 for in vivo Gene Therapy: Promise and Hurdles - Scientific Figure on Research Gate. Available from: https://www.researchgate.net/figure/Schematic-representation-of-CRISPR-Cas9-mediated-genome-editing-a-Schematic-of-CRISPR_fig1_308453321

[10] Esrick EB, Manis JP, Daley H, Baricordi C, Trebeden-Negre H, Pierciey FJ, et al. Successful hematopoietic stem cell mobilization and apheresis collection using plerixafor alone in sickle cell patients. Blood Advances. 2018;**2**:2505-2512. DOI: 10.1182/bloodadvances.2018016725

[11] Fitzhugh CD, Abraham AA, Tisdale JF, Hsieh MM. Hematopoietic stem cell transplantation for patients with sickle cell disease: Progress and future directions. Hematology/oncology Clinics of North America. 2014;**28**:1171-1185. DOI: 10.1016/j.hoc.2014.08.014

[12] Eggleston B, Patience M, Edwards S, Adamkiewicz T, Buchanan GR, Davies SC, et al. Effect of myeloablative bone marrow transplantation on growth in children with sickle cell anaemia: Results of the multicentre study of haematopoietic cell transplantation for sickle cell anaemia. British Journal of Haematology. 2007;**136**:673-676

[13] Bernaudin F, Socie G, Kuentz M, Chevret S, Duval M, Bertrand Y, et al. Long-term results of related myeloablative stem-cell transplantation to cure sickle cell disease. Blood. 2007;**110**:2749-2756

[14] O'Donnell PV, Luznik L, Jones RJ, Vogelsang GB, Leffell MS, Phelps M,

et al. Non-myeloablative bone marrow transplantation from partially HLA-mismatched related donors using post-transplantation cyclophosphamide. Biology of Blood and Marrow Transplantation. 2002;**8**:377-386

[15] Matthes-Martin S, Lawitschka A, Fritsch G, Lion T, Grimm B, Breuer S, et al. Stem cell transplantation after reduced-intensity conditioning for sickle cell disease. European Journal of Haematology. 2013;**90**:308-312

[16] Gluckman E, Cappelli B, Bernaudin F, Labopin M, Volt F, Carreras J, et al. Sickle cell disease: An international survey of results of HLA-identical sibling hematopoietic stem cell transplantation. Blood. 2016;**129**(11):1548-1556. DOI: 10.1182/blood-2016-10-745711

[17] Walters MC, Hardy K, Edwards S, Adamkiewicz T, Barkovich J, Bernaudin F, et al. Pulmonary, gonadal, and central nervous system status after bone marrow transplantation for sickle cell disease. Biology of Blood and Marrow Transplantation. 2010;**16**:263-272

[18] Vermylen C, Cornu G, Ferster A, Brichard B, Niane J, Ferrant A, et al. Haematopoietic stem cell transplantation for sickle cell anaemia: The first 50 patients transplanted in Belgium. Bone Marrow Transplantation. 1998;**22**:1-6

[19] Ola BA, Yates SJ, Dyson SM. Living with sickle cell disease and depression in Lagos, Nigeria: A mixed methods study. Social Science & Medicine. 2016;**161**:27-36. DOI: 10.1016/j.socscimed.2016.05.029

[20] Powars DR, Chan LS, Hiti A, Ramicone E, Johnson C. Outcome of sickle cell anaemia: A 4-decade observational study of 1056 patients. Medicine. 2005;**84**:363-376

[21] Walters MC, De Castro LM, Sullivan KM, Krishnamurti L, Kamani N, Bredeson C, et al. Indications and results of HLA-identical sibling hematopoietic cell transplantation for sickle cell disease. Biology of Blood and Marrow Transplantation. 2016;**22**:207-211

[22] Leonard A, Tisdale J, Abraham A. Curative options for sickle cell disease: Haploidentical stem cell transplantation or gene therapy? British Journal of Haematology. 2020;**189**(3):408-423. DOI: 10.1111/bjh.16437

[23] CSDH. Closing the Gap in a Generation: Health Equity through Action on the Social Determinants of Health. Final Report of the Commission on Social Determinants of Health. Geneva: World Health Organization; 2008

[24] Berghs M, Atkin K, Hatton C, et al. Rights to social determinants of flourishing? A paradigm for disability and public health research and policy. BMC Public Health. 2019;**19**:997. DOI: 10.1186/s12889-019-7334-8

[25] Gr D, Whitehead M. WHO. Levelling up (Part 2): A Discussion Paper on European Strategies for Tackling Social Inequities in Health/by Göran Dahlgren and Margaret WHitehead. Copenhagen: WHO Regional Office for Europe; 2006

[26] Sins JWR, Mager DJ, Davis S, Biemond BJ, Fijnvandraat K. Pharmacotherapeutical strategies in the prevention of acute, vaso-occlusive pain in sickle cell disease: A systematic review. Blood Advances. 2017;**1**:1598-1616. DOI: 10.1182/bloodadvances.2017007211

[27] Hsieh MM, Kang EM, Fitzhugh CD, Link B, Bolan CD, Kurlander R, et al. Allogeneic hematopoietic stem-cell transplantation for sickle cell disease. The New England Journal of Medicine. 2009;**361**:2309-2317

[28] Walters MC, Patience M, Leisenring W, Eckman JR, Buchanan GR, Rogers ZR, et al. Barriers to bone marrow transplantation for sickle cell anaemia. Biology of Blood and Marrow Transplantation. 1996;**2**:100-104

[29] Dallas MH, Triplett B, Shook DR, Hartford C, Srinivasan A, Laver J, et al. Long-term outcome and evaluation of organ function in paediatric patients undergoing haploidentical and matched related hematopoietic cell transplantation for sickle cell disease. Biology of Blood and Marrow Transplantation. 2013;**19**:820-830

[30] Walters MC, Patience M, Leisenring W, Rogers ZR, Aquino VM, Buchanan GR, et al. Stable mixed hematopoietic chimerism after bone marrow transplantation for sickle cell anaemia. Biology of Blood and Marrow Transplantation. 2001;**7**:665-673

[31] Pareek M, Bangash MN, Pareek N, et al. Ethnicity and COVID-19: An urgent public health research priority. Lancet. 2020;**395**:1421-1422. DOI: 10.1016/S0140-6736(20)30922-3

[32] Modell B, Darlison M. Global epidemiology of haemoglobin disorders and derived service indicators. Bulletin of the World Health Organization. 2008;**86**:480-487. DOI: 10.2471/BLT.06.036673

[33] Grosse SD, Odame I, Atrash HK, et al. Sickle cell disease in Africa: A neglected cause of early childhood mortality. American Journal of Preventive Medicine. 2011;**41**:S398-S405. DOI: 10.1016/j.amepre.2011.09.013

[34] WHO. Sickle-Cell Disease: A Strategy for the WHO African Region. Malabo, Equatorial Guinea: World Health Organization; 2011

[35] Burnham-Marusich AR, Ezeanolue CO, Obiefune MC, et al. Prevalence of sickle cell trait and reliability of self-reported status among expectant parents in Nigeria: Implications for targeted new born screening. Public Health Genomics. 2016;**19**:298-306. DOI: 10.1159/000448914

[36] Tluway F, Makani J. Sickle cell disease in Africa: An overview of the integrated approach to health, research, education and advocacy in Tanzania, 2004-2016. British Journal of Haematology. 2017;**177**(6):919-929

[37] Chakravorty SAK, Dziwinski S, Kaya B, et al. Optimising the transition from paediatric to adult care model for people with sickle cell disease – A UK multidisciplinary consensus statement. Health Sciences Journal. 2019;**13**:1-10

[38] Gragert L, Eapen M, Williams E, Freeman J, Spellman S, Baitty R, et al. HLA match likelihoods for hematopoietic stem-cell grafts in the U.S. registry. The New England Journal of Medicine. 2014;**371**:339-348

[39] Dyson SM. "Race", ethnicity and haemoglobin disorders. Social Science & Medicine. Jul 1998;**47**(1):121-131. DOI: 10.1016/s0277-9536(98)00023-9

[40] Gardner K, Douiri A, Drasar E, Allman M, Mwirigi A, Awogbade M, et al. Survival in adults with sickle cell disease in a high-income setting. Blood. 2016;**128**:1436-1438. DOI: 10.1182/blood-2016-05-716910

[41] Telen MJ, Malik P, Vercellotti GM. Therapeutic strategies for sickle cell disease: Towards a multi-agent approach. Nature Reviews. Drug Discovery. 2019;**18**:139-158. DOI: 10.1038/s41573-018-0003-2

[42] Sparkenbaugh E, Pawlinski R. Interplay between coagulation and

vascular inflammation in sickle cell disease. British Journal of Haematology. 2013;**162**:3-14. DOI: 10.1111/bjh.12336

[43] Nur E, Brandjes DP, Teerlink T, Otten HM, Oude Elferink RP, Muskiet F, et al. N-acetylcysteine reduces oxidative stress in sickle cell patients. Annals of Hematology. 2012;**91**:1097-1105. DOI: 10.1007/s00277-011-1404-z

[44] Telen MJ, Batchvarova M, Shan S, Bovee-Geurts PH, Zennadi R, Leitgeb A, et al. Sevuparin binds to multiple adhesive ligands and reduces sickle red blood cell-induced vaso-occlusion. British Journal of Haematology. 2016;**175**:935-948. DOI: 10.1111/bjh.14303

[45] Adegoke SA, Oladimeji OI, Ologun BG, Aladekomo TA, Oyelami OA. Outcome of short-term emergency department observation care of children with sickle cell disease and vaso-occlusive crises: Initial experience from South-Western Nigeria. Transactions of the Royal Society of Tropical Medicine and Hygiene. 2020;**114**:365-371. DOI: 10.1093/trstmh/traa006

[46] Adewoye AH, Nolan V, McMahon L, Ma Q, Steinberg MH. Effectiveness of a dedicated day hospital for management of acute sickle cell pain. Haematologica. 2007;**92**(6):854-855. DOI: 10.3324/haematol.10757

[47] Wright J, Bareford D, Wright C, Augustine G, Olley K, Musamadi L, et al. Day case management of sickle pain: 3 years' experience in a UK sickle cell unit. British Journal of Haematology. 2004;**126**(6):878-880. DOI: 10.1111/j.1365-2141.2004.05123.x

[48] Haywood C Jr et al. The impact of race and disease on sickle cell patient wait times in the emergency department. The American Journal of Emergency Medicine. 2013;**31**(4):651-656

[49] Glassberg JA et al. Emergency provider analgesic practices and attitudes towards patients with sickle cell disease. The American Journal of Emergency Medicine. 2013;**62**(4):293-302

[50] Shah N et al. Sickle cell disease complications: Prevalence and resource utilization. PLoS One. 2019;**14**(7):e0214355

[51] Elmariah H, Garrett ME, De Castro LM, Jonassaint JC, Ataga KI, Eckman JR, et al. Factors associated with survival in a contemporary adult sickle cell disease cohort. American Journal of Hematology. 2014;**89**:530-535. DOI: 10.1002/ajh.23683

[52] Tewari S, Brousse V, Piel FB, Menzel S, Rees DC. Environmental determinants of severity in sickle cell disease. Haematologica. 2015;**100**:1108-1116

[53] McGann PT. Sickle cell anaemia: An underappreciated and unaddressed contributor to global childhood mortality. The Journal of Pediatrics. 2014;**165**:18-22. DOI: 10.1016/j.jpeds.2014.01.070

[54] Adegoke SA, Akinlosotu MA, Adediji OB, Oyelami OA, Adeodu OO, Adekile AD. Sickle cell disease in Southwestern Nigeria: Assessment of knowledge of primary health care workers and available facilities. Transactions of the Royal Society of Tropical Medicine and Hygiene. 2018;**112**:81-87. DOI: 10.1093/trstmh/try025

[55] Ullrich H et al. Erythrocytapheresis: Do not forget a useful therapy! Transfusion Medicine and Hemotherapy. 2008;**35**(1):24-30

[56] Heeney MM, Hoppe CC, Abboud MR, Inusa B, Kanter J, Ogutu B, et al. A multinational trial of prasugrel for sickle cell vaso-occlusive events.

The New England Journal of Medicine. 2016;**374**:625-635. DOI: 10.1056/NEJMoa1512021

[57] Hoppe C, Jacob E, Styles L, Kuypers F, Larkin S, Vichinsky E. Simvastatin reduces vaso-occlusive pain in sickle cell anaemia: A pilot efficacy trial. British Journal of Haematology. 2017;**177**:620-629. DOI: 10.1111/bjh.14580

[58] The Lancet Haematology. CRISPR-Cas9 gene editing for patients with haemoglobinopathies. Lancet Haematology. 2019;**6**:E438

[59] Vakulskas CA, Dever DP, Rettig GR, Turk R, Jacobi AM, Collingwood MA, et al. A high-fidelity Cas9 mutant delivered as a ribonucleoprotein complex enables efficient gene editing in human hematopoietic stem and progenitor cells. Nature Medicine. 2018;**24**:1216-1224

[60] Urbinati F, Hargrove PW, Geiger S, Romero Z, Wherley J, Kaufman ML, et al. Potentially therapeutic levels of anti-sickling globin gene expression following lentivirus-mediated gene transfer in sickle cell disease bone marrow CD34+ cells. Experimental Hematology. 2015;**43**:346-351

[61] Ingram VM. Gene mutations in human haemoglobin: The chemical difference between normal and sickle cell haemoglobin. Nature. 1957;**180**:326-328

[62] Hoban MD, Lumaquin D, Kuo CY, Romero Z, Long J, Ho M, et al. CRISPR/Cas9-mediated correction of the sickle mutation in human CD34+ cells. Molecular Therapy. 2016;**24**:1561-1569

[63] Lattanzi A, Meneghini V, Pavani G, Amor F, Ramadier S, Felix T, et al. Optimization of CRISPR/Cas9 delivery to human hematopoietic stem and progenitor cells for therapeutic genomic rearrangements. Molecular Therapy. 2019;**27**:137-150

[64] Adams RJ et al. Long-term stroke risk in children with sickle cell disease screened with transcranial Doppler. Annals of Neurology. 1997;**42**(5):699-704

[65] Adams RJ et al. Transcranial Doppler correlation with cerebral angiography in sickle cell disease. Stroke. 1992;**23**(8):1073-1077

[66] Hassell KL. Sickle cell disease: A continued call to action. American Journal of Preventive Medicine. 2016;**51**:S1-S2. DOI: 10.1016/j.amepre.2015.11.002

[67] Silva-Pinto AC et al. Clinical and hematological effects of hydroxyurea therapy in sickle cell patients: A single-center experience in Brazil. São Paulo Medical Journal. 2013;**131**(4):238-243

[68] Brittenham GM, Schechter AN, Noguchi CT. Haemoglobin S polymerization: Primary determinant of the haemolytic and clinical severity of the sickling syndromes. Blood. 1985;**65**:183-189

[69] Eaton WA, Bunn HF. Treating sickle cell disease by targeting HbS polymerization. Blood. 2017;**129**:2719-2726. DOI: 10.1182/blood-2017-02-765891

[70] Berthaut I, Guignedoux G, Kirsch-Noir F, de Larouziere V, Ravel C, Bachir D, et al. Influence of sickle cell disease and treatment with hydroxyurea on sperm parameters and fertility of human males. Haematologica. 2008;**93**:988-993. DOI: 10.3324/haematol.11515

[71] Jain D et al. Sickle cell disease and pregnancy. Mediterranean Journal of Hematology and Infectious Diseases. 2019;**11**(1):e2019040

[72] Opoka RO, Ndugwa CM, Latham TS, Lane A, Hume HA, Kasirye P, et al. Novel use of hydroxyurea in an African region with malaria (NOHARM): A trial

for children with sickle cell anaemia. Blood. 2017;**130**:2585-2593. DOI: 10.1182/blood-2017-06-788935

[73] Cokic VP, Smith RD, Beleslin-Cokic BB, Njoroge JM, Miller JL, Gladwin MT, et al. Hydroxyurea induces foetal haemoglobin by the nitric oxide-dependent activation of soluble guanylyl cyclase. The Journal of Clinical Investigation. 2003;**111**:231-239. DOI: 10.1172/JCI16672

[74] Ware RE. Optimizing hydroxyurea therapy for sickle cell anemia. Hematology: the American Society of Hematology Education Program. 2015;**2015**:436-443. DOI: 10.1182/asheducation-2015.1.436

[75] McGann PT, Ware RE. Hydroxyurea therapy for sickle cell anaemia. Expert Opinion on Drug Safety. 2015;**14**(11):1749-1758

[76] Negre O, Bartholomae C, Beuzard Y, Cavazzana M, Christiansen L, Courne C, et al. Preclinical evaluation of efficacy and safety of an improved lentiviral vector for the treatment of β-thalassemia and sickle cell disease. Current Gene Therapy. 2015;**15**:64-81

[77] Angelucci E, Matthes-Martin S, Baronciani D, Bernaudin F, Bonanomi S, Cappellini MD, et al. Hematopoietic stem cell transplantation in thalassemia major and sickle cell disease: Indications and management recommendations from an international expert panel. Haematologica. 2014;**99**:811-820. DOI: 10.3324/haematol.2013.099747

[78] Gluckman E, Cappelli B, Bernaudin F, Labopin M, Volt F, Carreras J, et al. Sickle cell disease: An international survey of results of HLA-identical sibling hematopoietic stem cell transplantation. Blood. 2017;**129**:1548-1556. DOI: 10.1182/blood-2016-10-745711

[79] Joseph JJ, Abraham AA, Fitzhugh CD. When there is no match, the game is not over: Alternative donor options for hematopoietic stem cell transplantation in sickle cell disease. Seminars in Hematology. 2018;**55**:94-101. DOI: 10.1053/j.seminhematol.2018.04.013

[80] Johnson FL. Bone marrow transplantation in the treatment of sickle cell anaemia. The American Journal of Pediatric Hematology/Oncology. 1985;**7**:254-257

[81] Ataga KI, Kutlar A, Kanter J, Liles D, Cancado R, Friedrisch J, et al. Crizanlizumab for the prevention of pain crises in sickle cell disease. The New England Journal of Medicine. 2017;**376**:429-439. DOI: 10.1056/NEJMoa1611770

[82] Kutlar A, Kanter J, Liles DK, Alvarez OA, Cancado RD, Friedrisch JR, et al. Effect of crizanlizumab on pain crises in subgroups of patients with sickle cell disease: A SUSTAIN study analysis. American Journal of Hematology. 2019;**94**:55-61. DOI: 10.1002/ajh.25308

[83] Chinyakata R, Roman NV, Msiza FB. Stakeholders' perspectives on the barriers to accessing health care services in rural settings: A human capabilities approach. Open Public Health Journal. 2021;**14**:336-344. DOI: 10.2174/1874944502114010336

[84] Culyer AJ. Involving stakeholders in healthcare decisions: The experience of the national institute for clinical excellence (NICE) in England and Wales. Healthcare Quarterly. 2005;**8**(3):56-60. DOI: 10.12927/hcq.17155

[85] National Population Commission (Nigeria) and ICF. Nigeria Demographic and Health Survey 2018. Abuja and Rockville: National Population Commission (Nigeria) and ICF. Available from: https://dhsprogram.com/pubs/

pdf/FR359/FR359.pdf; 2019 [Accessed: November 19, 2019]

[86] Nnodu O. Interventions for the prevention and control of sickle cell disease at primary health care centres in Gwagwalada area Council of the Federal Capital Territory, Nigeria. Cureus. 2014;**6**(8):e194. DOI: 10.7759/cureus.194

[87] The federal ministry of health. National Guideline for the Control and Management of Sickle Cell Disease. Nigeria: The federal ministry of health; 2014. Available from: http://www.health.gov.ng/doc/SCDGuideline.pdf

[88] Piel FB, Hay SI, Gupta S, Weatherall DJ, Williams TN. Global burden of sickle cell anaemia in children under five, 2010-2050: Modelling based on demographics, excess mortality, and interventions. PLoS Medicine. 2013;**10**:e1001484. DOI: 10.1371/journal.pmed.1001484

Chapter 5

Screening of Newborn with Sickle Cell Disease in the View of Resource-Limited Setting

Runyararo Mashingaidze Mano

Abstract

Sickle cell disease (SCD) is a genetic hemoglobinopathy and has its highest prevalence in sub-Saharan Africa. It has contributed significantly to the morbidity and mortality in children under 5 years. In developed countries, newborn screening (NBS) followed by comprehensive care and community involvement have reduced SCD-related deaths by 10-fold. The life expectancy of SCD patients has also improved. Current practices in most resource-limited settings are mainly based on diagnosing symptomatic children upon presentation to health facilities. However, some countries in these settings have started introducing NBS. The common screening methods being used include high-performance liquid chromatography and isoelectric focusing. Despite some progress made in NBS, there have been some challenges. Some of these include the cost of screening, lack of qualified personnel, and the turnaround time for the results. In order to improve the care of children with SCD in resource-limited settings, there is a need to move toward point-of-care testing.

Keywords: sickle cell, resource limited, practice, newborn, screening

1. Introduction

Sickle cell disease (SCD) is a monogenic disorder with a complex genotype–phenotype correlation, influenced by both genetic and environmental factors [1, 2]. The disease is characterized by a mutation in the β-globin gene, leading to the substitution of valine for glutamic acid [3]. The clinical diversity of SCD is influenced by genomic polymorphisms, including coinheritance of α-thalassemia and haplotypes in the β-globin gene cluster [2]. These genetic modifiers, such as fetal hemoglobin concentration and α-thalassemia, play a significant role in the disease's severity and clinical manifestations [1, 3]. Understanding these genetic factors is crucial for predicting disease severity, guiding therapeutic interventions, and improving genetic counseling and prenatal diagnosis [1].

Sickle cell disease (SCD) is a significant global health concern, particularly prevalent in sub-Saharan Africa, the Mediterranean, the Middle East, and India [4]. Its incidence is increasing due to global migration, and it has been recognized as a public health problem by the World Health Organization [5].

IntechOpen

It affects approximately 5% of the world's population, with varying estimates across continents [6]. The prevalence of sickle cell disease in newborn populations in developing countries, such as Nigeria, remains high, highlighting the need for further progress in early diagnosis in these regions [7]. A systematic analysis of the burden of SCD over 21 years from 2000 to 2021 has shown an annual increase in the incidence of SCD by 13.7% to 515,000 cases in 2021. Additionally, the prevalence of SCD increased by 41.4% globally from 5.46 million in 2000 to 7.4 million in 2021 [6]. The majority of children born with SCD (50–90%) dies before their 5th birthday, approximately 150,000–300,000 annually in Africa. This potentially accounts for 5–10% of the region's total child mortality [6, 8, 9]. The disease is associated with a range of clinical complications, and there is a need for cost-effective diagnosis and efficient health interventions [10].

Early detection of sickle cell disease through newborn screening (NBS) is imperative. The main goal of NBS is to detect congenital disease in pre-symptomatic infants so that treatment may be commenced as early as possible to prevent, or ameliorate, the long-term consequences of the condition [11]. For a disease to be considered for NBS, it should meet the Wilson and Jungner criteria [12, 13]:

1. The condition sought should be an important health problem.
2. There should be an accepted treatment for patients with recognized disease.
3. Facilities for diagnosis and treatment should be available.
4. There should be a recognizable latent or early symptomatic stage.
5. There should be a suitable test or examination.
6. The test should be acceptable to the population.
7. The natural history of the condition, including development from latent to declared disease, should be adequately understood.
8. There should be an agreed policy on which to treat patients.
9. The cost of case-finding (including diagnosis and treatment of patients diagnosed) should be economically balanced in relation to possible expenditure on medical care as a whole.
10. Case-finding should be a continuous process and not a "once and for all" project [12, 13].

In developed countries, newborn screening (NBS) for SCD among under-5 children has been shown to improve their survival and also reduce mortality by 10 folds due to interventions done before development of complications [10]. In England, for example, the implementation of the screening program resulted in the identification of a high number of carriers and those with SCD [14]. Results from this study were further supported by another study by Shook in the USA [15], which emphasized the effectiveness of newborn screening in improving child health.

2. Evolution of sickle cell disease newborn screening

Sickle cell disease was first described in 1910 by Herrick and Irons, who observed the irregularly shaped blood cells in a 32-year-old dental student, Walter Clement Noel, who died suddenly after presenting with joint pain and shortness of breath [16, 17]. He was a native of Grenada and had just returned home after graduation [16, 17]. The discovery of the abnormal red blood cells was groundbreaking in medical history, and this led to a deeper understanding of the disease, its clinical features, and pathophysiology. It also paved the way for further research into the molecular characteristics and behavior of sickle hemoglobin [18]. Moreover, it was later confirmed to be caused by an autosomal recessive inherited hemoglobinopathy, the gene responsible for the transmission of the disease being introduced into the new world during the 17th century [19, 20]. This was further clarified in 1949 by Pauling and his associates, who identified the abnormal hemoglobin (Hb) responsible for the sickling phenomenon. Neel and Beet further described the inheritance of the disease [20]. The confirmation of the autosomal recessive nature of sickle cell disease has been a significant milestone in understanding and managing this condition [21].

The foundation of newborn screening stems from the work of Robert Guthrie, a microbiologist who had a disabled child initially thought to be due to phenylketonuria (PKU), although he tested negative [22]. This discovery led to massive and rapid screening of children with similar clinical features. Over the years, more and more diseases, including PKU, hypothyroidism, galactosemia, and congenital adrenal hyperplasia, have been added to list of newborn screening in many parts of the developed world [11]. Concerning sickle cell disease NBS, it was not until the early 1970s that some form of sickle cell screening was introduced in the Unites States of America following pressure from the African American Advocacy groups [23]. New York piloted universal newborn screening program in 1975, with the rest of the states adopting the screening throughout the late 1990s and into 2000s. The initial screening programs targeted at-risk populations, primarily African Americans. However, this resulted in 30% of cases being missed, which resulted in the introduction of universal screening [24].

Prior to NBS, sickle cell disease was diagnosed in symptomatic individuals using blood films, solubility, and sickling test. A study at Makerere University of Health Sciences in Uganda was carried out to determine the reliability of sickling and solubility tests and peripheral blood film method for screening for SCD [25]. The study reported that peripheral blood smear (PBF) had a sensitivity of 35.0%, specificity of 96.7%, and accuracy of 90.5%. It had simple preparation and a turnaround time (TAT) of 44 minutes and was inexpensive [25]. Unfortunately, the test depends on the pathologist's skills and does not differentiate between different types of SCD [25]. It detects sickle cells which are usually absent in the new born due to high levels of fetal hemoglobin (HbF) [26]. Solubility was noted to have a sensitivity of 65%, specificity of 90.0%, and accuracy of 85% [25]. In contrast, sickling had a sensitivity 45.0%, specificity 95.6%, and accuracy of 92.5% [25]. Both tests are easy, inexpensive, fast, and affordable, with TAT of 38 minutes for sickling and 70 minutes for solubility. Testing newborns shows false-negative result, does not differentiate between SCD types, and only detects sickling events [25].

Technical advancements in laboratory methods for sickle cell disease detection have also been achieved in developed countries [27]. The laboratory method employed for screening was the citrate agar electrophoresis using cord blood and later heel stick samples (dried blood spot) [27]. Currently in developed countries, a majority of hemoglobinopathy NBS programs use the combination of isoelectric focusing (IEF) and high-performance liquid chromatography (HPLC) as primary screening methods [23]. However, traditional laboratory-based screening methods may not be feasible in resource-constrained settings. As such, point-of-care tests (POCTs) offer a promising alternative for SCD newborn screening in such settings [28].

3. Current NBS in resource-limited settings

In resource-limited settings, NBS programs are yet to be established fully. Some countries have introduced NBS as part of research. Major screening programs have started in parts of Uganda, Tanzania, Nigeria, Haiti, and India [29–33]. Different laboratory methods were used for screening, the main ones being laboratory based.

3.1 Traditional laboratory methods

Traditional laboratory methods used so far include:

High-performance liquid chromatography [34]: It uses the principles of cation exchange for the separation and determination of the relative percentage of normal and abnormal hemoglobin (Hb) [35]. Additionally, HPLC separates hemoglobin in sample by passing them through a column filled with a solid adsorbent material [36]. Each component in the sample interacts slightly differently with the adsorbent material, causing different flow rates for different components and leading to the separation of the components as they flow out the column [35]. This is the method used to identify and quantify relative fractions of Hb F, Hb A2, Hb S, Hb C, Hb Barts, and other Hb variants. HPLC is also used to quantify Hb A2 and Hb F for carrier screening [37]. However, there is a chance of misdiagnosing the new variants that mimic HbS. It is expensive and needs trained personnel and may not be practical in resource-limited areas.

Isoelectric focusing (IEF) [38]: It utilizes agarose gels to separate hemoglobin (Hb) fractions and variants based on their isoelectric points. Hb A and Hb F are clearly resolved by this method [39]. Hb C can also be distinguished from Hb E and Hb O, and Hb S can be distinguished from Hb. Detects HbS and HbA easily even in a high concentration of HbF. HbDPunjab can easily be separated from HbS. A small volume of blood is needed and dried blood spot samples can be used. It has a turnaround time (TAT) of 45 minutes [39]. However, it is expensive and requires highly trained staff to interpret the results [39].

Electrophoresis [40]: Hemoglobin electrophoresis either at acidic or alkaline pH can be used as a primary or confirmatory method of identification [35]. Hemoglobin is separated into bands based on mobility of the variant and charge. It is reliable and has the ability to distinguish most types of sickle cell disease including heterozygous [39]. The electrophoresis can identify and quantify HbF, Hb A, Hb A2, Hb S, Hb C, Hb Barts, and others. However, it is expensive and requires skilled technicians [39].

Deoxyribonucleic acid (DNA) analysis Polymerase chain Reaction (PCR): This test requires special enzymes to amplify specific parts of the genetic materials to millions using specific primers. PCR can detect well-known single genes or several genes in a single tube [39]. The PCR program involves denaturation, annealing, and elongation, which is repeated for 20 to 40 thermal cycles [39]. Afterward the results are detected by gel electrophoresis, sequencing, or melting curve analysis or monitoring the change in the florescence [39]. Melting curve analysis or high-resolution melting (HRM), which is simple, sensitive, and cost effective for mass screening of SCD genotypes, detects β_S mutations [41]. Another low-cost, simple PCR-based technique has been developed using bidirectional allele-specific amplification (ASA) and a hot star system to provide more specific single-tube genotyping where the point mutation of sickle cell anemia is used as single nucleotide polymorphism (SNP) [42]. Another PCR technique, amplification refractory mutation system (ARMS), is considered to be simple for detecting point mutation or small deletion [43]. The ARMS principle uses primers with specific sequences to allow for amplification of DNA in the presence of the target allele. Hence, the detection of the target allele is based on the presence of the PCR product [43]. These PCR techniques mentioned above, although considered simple, are relatively expensive and require specialized personnel [39].

Restriction fragment length polymorphism (RFLP): RFLP is used to detect sickle cell disease based on restriction enzymes, which remove the recognition site at the β-mutated gene [44]. MtsII is one of the first described restriction enzymes (**Figure 1**) [39]. In homozygous, the enzyme cuts both genes, and two bands appear. In the sickle trait, (β AβS), no cut is made in the βS, so a single band appears, but the βA gene is cleaved, and two bands appear [39]. In sickle cell anemia homozygous (βSβS), there is no enzyme cutting due to the mutation in both genes, so a single wide band appears [39]. Another restriction enzyme used in sickle cell detection is Ddel. In this case, the enzyme removes the restriction site Ddel, 5'-GTNAG-3'. Bands with different lengths appear depending on the presence or absence of sickle cell anemia mutation [45]. A study by Ngole et al. in 2021 [46] from the Democratic Republic of Congo in newborn babies using RFLP reported a decrease in cost by half compared with IEF for sickle cell disease NBS. Despite this cost reduction, RFLP remains time consuming and expensive and requires experts in the area [39].

DNA microarray and sequencing techniques: DNA microarrays are designed with known DNA sequences that are specific to particular genes or regions of interest [47]. These probes are typically short sequences of single-stranded DNA [47]. The microarrays have been in genomic wide association studies (GWAS) used to identify SNPs [2]. Sanger sequencing, also known as the chain-termination method, is a technique used for DNA sequencing. It was developed by Frederick Sanger and his colleagues in 1977.

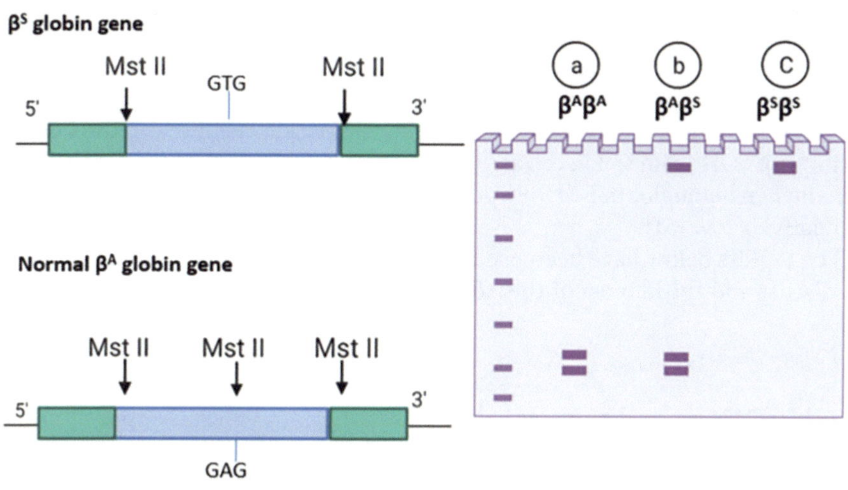

Figure 1.
Restriction fragment length polymorphism (RFLP) for sickle cell anemia: (a) normal gene (βAβA); (b) sickle cell trait (βAβS); and (c) sickle cell anemia (βSβS) [39].

In Sanger sequencing, DNA is replicated *in vitro* using a DNA polymerase enzyme, with the addition of modified nucleotides called dideoxynucleotides (ddNTPs) [47]. In resource-limited settings, Sanger sequencing was used for validation of laboratory methods for sickle cell disease NBS [48]. Next-generation sequencing (NGS) is a new technology used for DNA and RNA sequencing and variant/mutation detection [48]. The sequencing techniques help with precision medicine. However, the exorbitant cost and the need for qualified personnel limit the techniques to validation in a research set up in resource-limited settings [48].

The traditional laboratory methods' disadvantages

- Require trained personnel
- Equipment is expensive to purchase and maintain.
- May be limited to centralized laboratories, which may not be easily accessible
- Turnaround time is long.
- Difficult to implement on a large scale for resource-limited settings
- Consumables expensive

3.2 Point-of-care tests

Point-of-care tests (POCT), which provide timely results needed for prompt management, have revolutionized the diagnosis of sickle cell disease in developing countries [49]. According to the World Health Organization, an ideal diagnostic point-of-care test (POCT) must be Affordable, Sensitive, Specific, User friendly, Rapid/Robust, Equipment free, and Deliverable (ASSURED) [50]. The ASSURED criteria represent three main attributes that are significant for a diagnostic test, which are accessibility, affordability, and accuracy [50]. The advancement of the digital age has led to a revision of the ASSURED criteria to REASSURED: Real-time connectivity, Ease of specimen collection, Affordable, Sensitive, Specific, User-friendly, Rapid and robust, Equipment-free or simple, and Deliverable to end-user (**Table 1**) [51]. Additionally, the POCT should strengthen healthcare systems, ensure system efficiency, and improve patient outcome [51]. For sickle cell disease, the POCT should distinguish SCD from sickle cell trait (SCT) and diagnostic accuracy in the newborn period when hemoglobin F (HbF) predominates and when hemoglobin S (HbS) levels are relatively low [51].

The POCTs below have been used in resource-limited settings for NBS for sickle cell disease and fulfill most of the ASSURED criteria.

3.2.1 SickleSCAN

SickleSCAN is a qualitative lateral flow immunoassay which uses polyclonal antibodies [52]. The kit is supplied as a cassette with tests and can be stored for up to two years at room temperature [52]. Sampling technique is by finger or heel prick and can be used on venous blood [52]. Sample reading is straightforward: positive results are seen as bands on the cassette, and minimum training is needed [52]. Turnaround time for the result: 3–5 min [53]. Bands do not fade on the cassette and are available for comparison

Real-time connectivity	Tests connected to reader or mobile phone
Ease of collection	Non-invasive specimens
Affordable	Affordable to end-users and health systems
Sensitive	Low false-negative rate
Specific	Low false-positive rate
User-friendly	Simple testing procedure with limited training
Rapid and Robust	Tests available at time of visit without additional transport or special storage conditions (within 15 min to 2 h)
Equipment-free and environmentally friendly	Ideally does not require special equipment or can be operated using battery or solar power
Delivered to those who will benefit	Accessible to those who need testing the most

Table 1.
Reassured criteria [11].

with the result of confirmatory testing [53]. It has a sensitivity (on-field conditions) of >94·9% [54] and specificity (on-field conditions) of >99·2% [54], with an overall diagnostic accuracy of 99%29 [55]. The average cost per test is US$2·19 to < US$ 5 [55].

3.2.2 HemoTypeSC

This is a competitive lateral flow assay incorporating monoclonal antibodies [28]. The kit is supplied as dipsticks in a test tube and is stable at room temperature [28]. Sampling technique is by finger or heel prick [28], and sample reading is counterintuitive: the absence of a band is the positive result, and rigorous training is needed [28]. It has a turnaround time of 10 minutes for the result [56]. The test has a sensitivity (on-field conditions) of >93·8% [57], specificity (on-field conditions) of >99·2% [57], and overall diagnostic accuracy of >99% [57]. HemotypeSC has an average cost per test of US$1·49 to < US$5 [57]. Even though the test strips can be mounted on paper with the results, they are available for comparison with the result of confirmatory testing for a limited period because the test strip paper shows a sign of fragmentation with time (**Figures 2** and **3**) [53, 54].

3.2.3 Microchip-based cellulose acetate electrophoresis test 'gazelle'

The test uses Hb electrophoresis on a much smaller machine, which can be used at the community level [59]. The device is operated by rechargeable lithium batteries

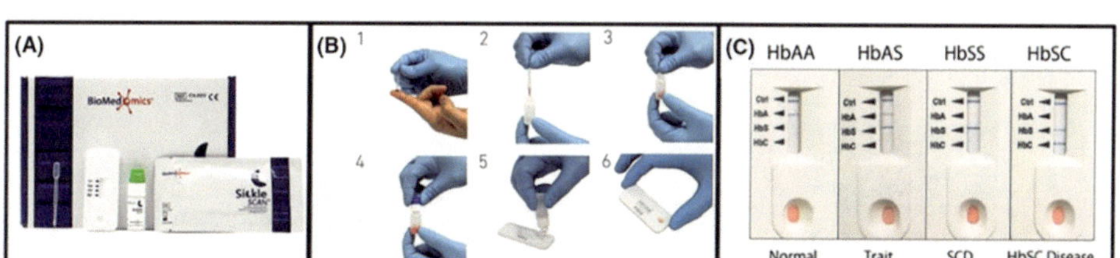

Figure 2.
SickleSCAN step by step [58].

that can test all day on a single charge [60] and also carries advanced features like WiFi, GPS, and Bluetooth-enabled connectivity for easy tracking of samples and can connect to a printer wirelessly [60]. The turnaround time is 8 minutes [60]. The test, however, requires skilled personnel to carry out and interpret (**Figure 4**).

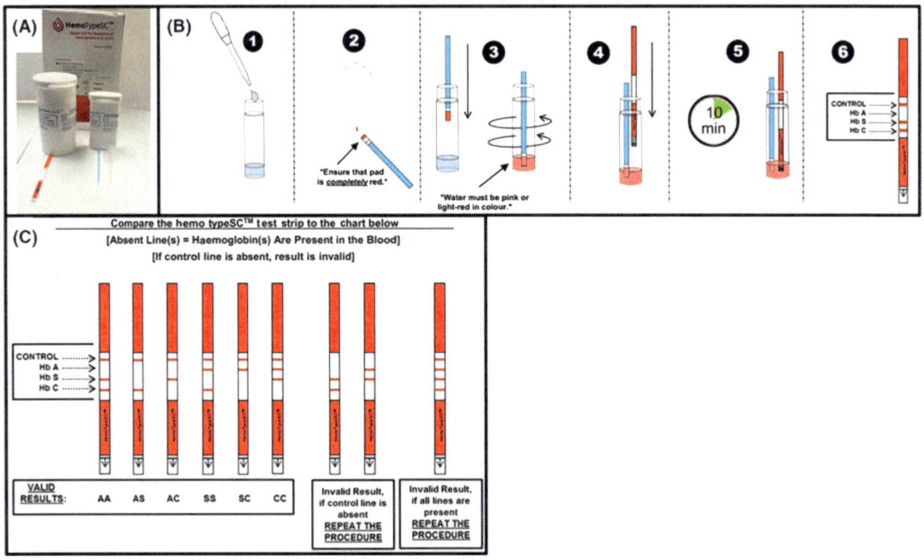

Figure 3.
HemotypeSC test step by step [58].

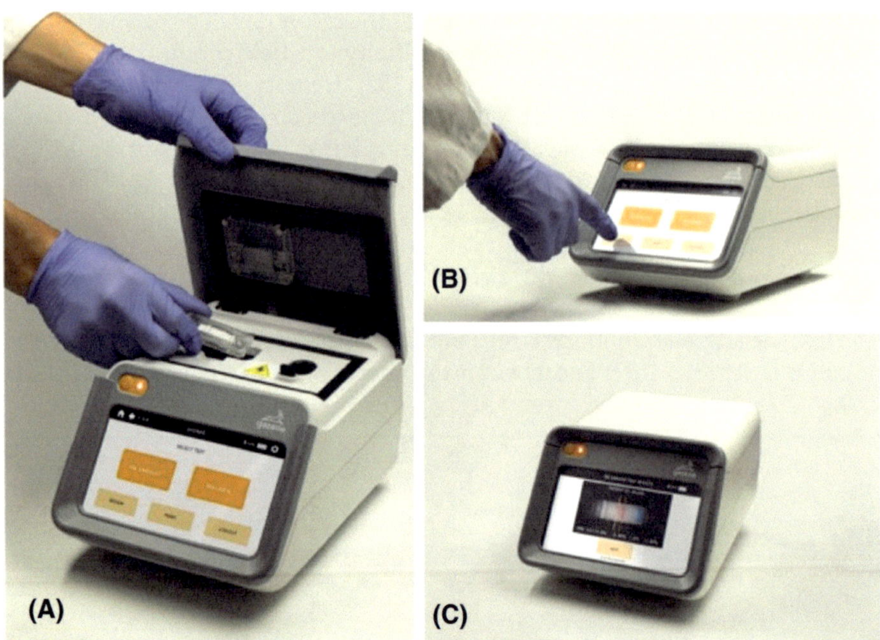

Figure 4.
Gazelle Hb variant [58].

Table 2 is adopted and summarizes the POCTs for sickle cell disease. It highlights studies that used the different screening tools and their sensitivity.

3.2.4 Other point-of-care tests

Paper-based Sickle test (microfluid assessment) (**Figure 5**) [64].

This screening method is inexpensive and requires non-skilled personnel [39]. TAT is approximately 20 minutes. It has a sensitivity of 94.25% (for detection of HbS presence) [65–67] and specificity of 97.7% (for detection of HbS presence) [65–67].

Test	HemoTypeSC	Sickle Scan	Gazelle Hb Variant
Technology	LFIA – Monoclonal abs to HbA, S, C	LFIA – Polyclonal abs to HbA, S, C	Modified cellulose acetate electrophoresis detecting Hb A, F, S C, E, A2
Time	10 min	5 min	8 min
Equipment	None	None	Requires electrical supply.
Field Validation	*Ghana* (n = 384) [61] Sensitivity: 100% Specificity: 100% *Nigeria* (n = 1121) [53] Sensitivity: 93·4% Specificity: 99·1% *Nigeria* (n = 3603) [62] Sensitivity: 100% Specificity: 100% *India* (n = 1559) [61] Sensitivity: 98·1% Specificity: 99·1%	*Haiti* (n = 1372) [57] Sensitivity: 90% Specificity: 97% *Tanzania* (n = 652) [32] Sensitivity: 98·7% Specificity: 92·6% *Mali* (n = 80) [28] Sensitivity: 100% Specificity: 100% *Togo* (n = 209) [28] Sensitivity: 94·9–100% (genotype dependent) Specificity: > 99·2%	*Nigeria* (n = 315) [63] Sensitivity: 100% Specificity: 98% *Nigeria, Thailand, India, USA* (n = 768) [63] Overall diagnostic accuracy: 98·4%
Strengths	Accurate in young infants with high HbF Competitive against gold standard Low cost Validated within the infant screening framework (Nigeria)	Accurate in young infants with high HbF Competitive against gold standard Low cost Validated within the infant screening framework (Haiti) Easy, intuitive result interpretation	Accurate in infants Can detect non-HbS, HbC variants Quantitation of HbF, HbS Automated results Digital upload and data storage Possible linkage to malaria and hemoglobin testing with the same machine
Limitations	Counterintuitive interpretation of results Limited to genotypes containing HbA, S, and C [geographical limitation] Unable to diagnose beta-thalassemia	Limited to genotypes containing HbA, S & C [geographical limitation] Weak HbA band	Requires validation in the NBS setting Requires moderately complex laboratory processing Currently unable to detect beta-thalassaemia variants Requires battery power/electrical supply

Table 2.
Summary of the Common POCTs for newborn screening for sickle cell disease (Adapted from Serving lives [58].

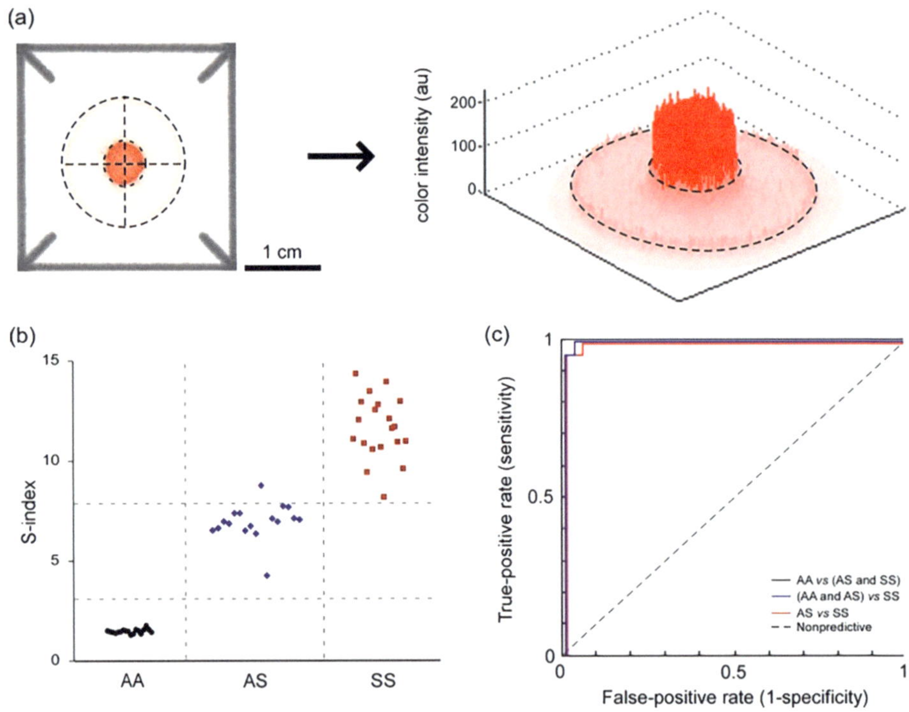

Figure 5.
Automated analysis of paper-based sickle test [39].

In terms of cost, the automated equipment cost US$ 300 to 500 [64]. Interpretation may be difficult as it requires a scanner for interpretation [35, 65]. The shortfall, however, cannot distinguish HbSC and HbAS. In addition, blood clotting interferes with the test [64], and the interpretation of results may be susceptible to human error [64].

HemeChip (Microengineered Electrophoresis) (**Figure 6**). It is reliable and able to distinguish most types of sickle cell disease including compound heterozygotes [64]. It is low cost and easy to use and has robustness and rapid testing [64]. The results for HemeChip are comparable to standard electrophoresis tests [64], Additionally, there is possible integration with mobile devices and works on principles of clinical standard electrophoresis [64]. Unfortunately, high HbF concentration present in newborns less than 4 weeks of age may affect test results. The cost per test is approximately US$0.9, with the cost of equipment being $500 (for automated detection) [39]. Its turnaround time (TAT) is less than 10 minutes, and it has a sensitivity of 89–100% [64] and specificity of 82–89% [64]. However, it requires skilled interpretation and is web-based and automated, and this is out of reach of most resource-limited regions [35].

Aqueous multiphase System (AMPS) (density-based test to separate Hb in different density fluids) (**Figure 6**) [35, 64].

It is a rapid test with a TAT of 10 minutes [64]. However, it needs batching for centrifuge operation, and this need for bulky centrifuges limits applicability to POC settings [64]. The other major drawback is its inability to distinguish between HbAA and HbAS [64]. Furthermore, inaccuracies are due to high HbF levels and health and

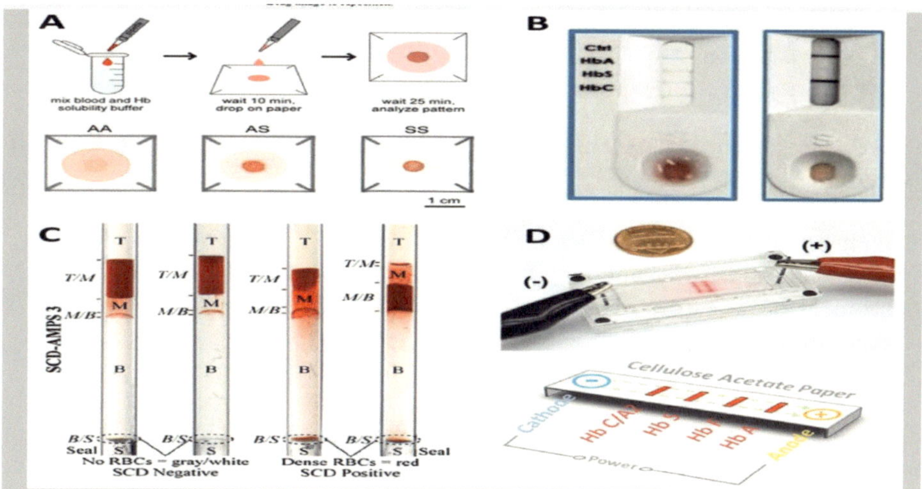

Figure 6.
Illustrations of emerging technologies in SCD [39]. "(A) Paper-based Hemoglobin solubility [68]. A droplet of blood mixed with Hb solubility buffer is dropped on chromatography paper, and a blood stain is allowed to form. The stain on paper is analyzed and the color intensity profiles are used to determine the Hb type in the sample. (B) Sickle Scan™ lateral flow immunoassay [55]. The test specimen consisting of a drop of blood mixed with Hb solubility buffer is dropped onto the sample loading zone. The solution then diffuses to the test zones where Hb is captured by color-conjugated antibodies. The type of Hb is determined by the appearance of a blue line at the different test zones along the test strip. (C) Density-based separation [69]. The blood sample is mixed with aqueous polymeric solutions in capillary tubes. Upon centrifugation, the precipitation of a dense RBC layer at the bottom of the tube indicates SCD. (D) Microengineered electrophoresis (HemeChip) [35]. After loading the blood sample mixed with DI water into the chip, an applied electric field causes Hb separation. Due to the differences in mobility among Hb types, each type will travel a unique distance across the paper strip".

treatment conditions, and genetic factors affect RBC density [64]. In addition, the equipment is expensive (cost US$150–1600) [64]. The sensitivity is 90–91% (for the identification of HbSS and HbSC with two-phase and three-phase AMPS) [64], and specificity is 88% [64].

4. Gaps in screening

Few countries have established SCD newborn screening programs in resource-limited settings, and research has identified significant gaps in resource-limited settings, particularly in sub-Saharan Africa. Conventional diagnostic methods are often cost-prohibitive and require specialized equipment and electricity, leading to delayed or missed diagnoses [67, 70]. Additionally, there is lack of qualified personnel, and laboratories are poorly resourced. The development of low-cost, rapid, and equipment-free paper-based tests and point-of-care diagnostics, like HemoTypeSC™, have shown promise in improving the practicality and accuracy of SCD screening in these settings [28, 67]. These innovations have the potential to reduce the overall cost of screening and increase the reach of universal newborn SCD screening programs. Other gaps include lack of awareness and regular monitoring of affected babies. Lack of policymakers' involvement, including financial commitments, is a major gap in the establishment of NBS programs [71]. Moreover, challenges in referral and follow-up persist, with delays in treatment. As a result, patients present with acute crisis, which is potentially prevented if babies are diagnosed early. Many a times, patients are lost to follow-up due to lack of proper follow-up guidelines [72].

5. Best practice for the establishment of NBS for SCD in resource-limited settings

Sickle cell disease newborn screening in low-resource settings can help identify affected infants early, allowing for timely intervention and management. Traditional laboratory methods are expensive and require skilled personnel. POCTs that meet the ASSURED/REASSURED criteria seem to be the best way to expand NBS for SCD in resource-limited settings [11]. However, implementing point-of-care tests for SCD in such settings requires a thoughtful approach to ensure effectiveness, affordability, and sustainability. Some of the best practices to put into consideration are:

5.1 Screening test selection

The choice of screening test should be based on the ASSURED/REASSURED criteria and be suitable for the local context. Additionally, it should be offered free of charge for families or made affordable [51]. Equally important, the test should be validated for use in the target population [51]

5.2 Community engagement

Community engagement is a crucial aspect of implementing newborn screening (NBS) for sickle cell disease (SCD) in sub-Saharan Africa [73, 74]. Community engagement is important to ensure local communities participate and that awareness about SCD, its inheritance pattern, and impact of early screening is raised [73, 74]. Equally important, there is a need for continuous multilevel evaluation by stakeholders, [73, 74]. In addition, community engagement promotes cultural sensitivity and addresses cultural beliefs and misconception, as well as the involvement of community leaders in program development cements the program [73, 74]. Engaging individuals with SCD in patient-centered research is also vital, as demonstrated by Mayo-Gamble in Tennessee in 2020 [75], who trained Community Health Ambassadors to serve as liaisons between researchers and the SCD community. In addition, individuals with sickle cell may identify research and management priorities. Lastly, a study by Hines [76] in 2011 presents a successful model for engaging patients and their families with SCD education, research, and community awareness. The above studies collectively underscore the importance of community engagement in NBS for SCD and provide valuable insights into its successful implementation.

5.3 Integration of NBS into existing health programs

Integrating SCD screening into existing maternal and child health programs helps to reach a wider community. In Tanzania, for instance, NBS was successfully integrated as part of the immunization program [53]. In Ghana, the integrated screening program resulted in the training of nurses and midwives [77]. The drawbacks with integration include inadequate nursing staff [77], shortage of screening supplies [77], and delay in receiving screening results (if traditional laboratory method is used rather than POCT) [77]. Successful integration requires partnership with program leaders, professionals, patients, and families. There is need to leverage resources from existing programs [71].

5.4 Stakeholder collaboration

Establishment of collaborative network for implementing and sustaining SCD newborn screening considers [78]: engagement of healthcare providers [78], government agencies [78], non-governmental organizations [78], community leaders, and resource-rich countries. International collaborations can lead to national guideline creation, improved clinical care, and research [78]. Full partnership, proper planning, and financial issues need to be addressed before program launch. In addition, rigorous program management is required to ensure its full effect and long sustainability [78].

5.5 Training and capacity building

Training of healthcare workers and community health volunteers to perform screening test and interpret results accurately is paramount [79, 80]. In the same vein, a sustainable training program for new personnel is required [79, 80]. In addition, training on proper counseling and support to families is needed [79, 80].

5.6 Sample collection and handling

There is need to develop standardized procedure for collection, labeling, and transporting of blood samples [67]. Furthermore, proper disposal of processed samples is required [67]. Equally important, challenges and solutions related to sample handling in resource-limited settings should be identified [67].

5.7 Quality control and assurance

Quality control and assurance include implementation of a rigorous quality control program to monitor and maintain accuracy and reliability of screening tests [28], ensuring expiry dates are documented and followed for testing [28] and regular calibration and maintenance of testing equipment where applicable [28].

5.8 Data management and record keeping

A successful program requires the review or design of systems for data management including patient record and test results [64]. Considering the use of technology and electronic records where feasible to be explored [64]. In addition, confidentiality of sensitive patient information by using secure and reliable data storage methods should be ensured [64].

5.9 Follow-up and referral system

A successful screening program requires the development of well-defined referral protocols for infants with positive screening results including confirmatory testing and access to specialized care and appropriate management [72]. In addition, it should ensure families understand the importance of follow-up care [72].

5.10 Counseling and support services

Provision of counseling and support services to families of infants diagnosed with SCD to help them understand the disease, manage/cope with its challenges, and access appropriate care and treatment is required [81]. Of equal importance is addressing any stigma and discrimination that may arise as a result of a positive result. In the same vein, culturally sensitive and effective training programs for counselors are of great importance [81]. The importance of early initiation of prophylactic therapy and parental education cannot be ignored [82].

5.11 Advocacy and policy influence

Government input is required for a successful screening program. The government should support and spearhead policy changes to integrate SCD screening into the national health system [71, 83]. Additionally, it must work toward securing funding for long-term sustainability of the program and avail funds for medicine and testing kits. It is important to note that the government is a key stakeholder involved in policy development and implementation [71, 83].

5.12 Monitoring and evaluation

Monitoring and evaluation are the backbone of any program. It is important to ensure that there is continuous monitoring and evaluation of program's performance including the number of infants screened [84], evaluation of positive cases identified and follow-up outcomes and use data to make improvements and adjustments as needed. Furthermore, evaluation of the effectiveness of training programs and ensuring accurate and consistent screening [84] form part of monitoring and evaluation. Assessment of key metrics tracked and the impact of screening on SCD diagnosis and management are needed [84].

6. Conclusion

Sickle cell disease can be a debilitating condition contributing significantly to morbidity and mortality worldwide. The World Health Organization estimates that 70% of SCD deaths in Africa can be preventable with simple, cost-effective interventions such as early identification of SCD patients by newborn screening and subsequent provision of comprehensive care. Much thought and commitment, including the choice of screening methods, have to be put into consideration prior to the establishment of newborn screening. Considerable efforts into development of point-of-care test have taken place over the years, and this move is likely to improve the coverage of SCD newborn screening program in resource-limited settings.

Author details

Runyararo Mashingaidze Mano
Faculty of Health Sciences and Veterinary Medicine, Department of Maternal and Child Health, Division of Paediatrics, School of Medicine, University of Namibia, Windhoek, Namibia

*Address all correspondence to: mashingaidzemano2003@gmail.com

References

[1] Thein SL. Genetic modifiers of sickle cell disease. Hemoglobin. 2011;**35** (5-6):589-606. DOI: 10.3109/03630269.2011.615876 Epub 2011 Oct 3

[2] Fertrin KY, Costa FF. Genomic polymorphisms in sickle cell disease: Implications for clinical diversity and treatment. Expert Review of Hematology. 2010;**3**(4):443-458. DOI: 10.1586/ehm.10.44

[3] Martin H. Steinberg BGF, Douglas R. Higgs and David J. Weatherall. Disorders of Hemoglobin Genetics, Pathophysiology, and Clinical Management. USA: Boston University; 2009. pp. 587-588. DOI: 10.1017/CBO9780511596582.032. [Accessed: March 1, 1978]

[4] Colombatti R, Birkegård C, Medici M. PB2215: Global epidemiology of sickle cell disease: A systematic literature review. HemaSphere. 2022;**6**:1. DOI: 10.1097/01.HS9.0000851688.00394.f4

[5] Mburu J, Odame I. Sickle cell disease: Reducing the global disease burden. International Journal of Laboratory Hematology. 2019;**41**(Suppl. 1):82-88. DOI: 10.1111/ijlh.13023

[6] Piel FB, Hay SI, Gupta S, Weatherall DJ, Williams TN. Global burden of sickle cell anaemia in children under five, 2010-2050: Modelling based on demographics, excess mortality, and interventions. PLOS Medicine. 2013;**10**(7):e1001484. DOI: 10.1371/journal.pmed.1001484 Epub 2013 Jul 16

[7] Odunvbun ME, Okolo AA, Rahimy CM. Newborn screening for sickle cell disease in a Nigerian hospital. Public Health. 2008;**122**(10):1111-1116. DOI: 10.1016/j.puhe.2008.01.008. Epub 2008 May 19

[8] Kato GJ, Piel FB, Reid CD, Gaston MH, Ohene-Frempong K, Krishnamurti L, et al. Sickle cell disease. Nature Reviews. Disease Primers. 2018;**4**:18010. DOI: 10.1038/nrdp.2018.10

[9] Thomson AM, McHugh TA, Oron AP, Teply C, Lonberg N, Vilchis Tella V, et al. Global, regional, and national prevalence and mortality burden of sickle cell disease, 2000-2021: A systematic analysis from the global burden of disease study 2021. The Lancet Haematology. 2023;**10**(8):e585-ee99

[10] Martinez RMO-AH, McCormick M. A strategic plan and blueprint for action: Complications of sickle cell disease and current management approaches. Available from: https://www.ncbi.nlm.nih.gov/books/NBK566466/. In: National Academies of Sciences E, and Medicine; Health and Medicine Division; Board on Population Health and Public Health Practice; Committee on Addressing Sickle Cell Disease: A Strategic Plan and Blueprint for Action. Washington (DC): National Academies Press (US): 2020 [Accessed: January 15, 2024]

[11] Pitt JJ. Newborn screening. Clinical Biochemist Reviews. 2010;**31**(2):57-68

[12] Andermann A, Blancquaert I, Beauchamp S, Déry V. Revisiting Wilson and Jungner in the genomic age: A review of screening criteria over the past 40 years. Bulletin of the World Health Organization. 2008;**86**(4):317-319. DOI: 10.2471/blt.07.050112

[13] World Health Organization, Wilson JMG, Jungner G. The Principles and Practice of Screening for Disease.

London and Sweden: World Health Organization; 1966. Available from: https://iris.who.int/handle/10665/208882

[14] Streetly A, Latinovic R, Hall K, Henthorn J. Implementation of universal newborn bloodspot screening for sickle cell disease and other clinically significant haemoglobinopathies in England: Screening results for 2005-7. Journal of Clinical Pathology. 2009;**62**(1):26-30. DOI: 10.1136/jcp.2008.058859

[15] Lisa MS, Russell EW. Effective screening leads to better outcomes in sickle cell disease. Archives of Disease in Childhood. 2018;**103**(7):628. ul;103(7):628-630. DOI: 10.1136/archdischild-2017-314175. Epub 2018 Feb 14

[16] Vichinsky EP. Pulmonary hypertension in sickle cell disease. The New England Journal of Medicine. 2004;**350**(9):857-859

[17] Serjeant GR. The emerging understanding of sickle cell disease. British Journal of Haematology. 2001;**112**(1):3-18. DOI: 10.1056/NEJMp038250

[18] Savitt TL, Goldberg MF. Herrick's 1910 case report of sickle cell anemia. The Rest of the Story. Jama. 1989;**261**(2):266-271

[19] Singh} MKDCaM. An Overview on Sickle Cell Disease Profile. Medicne. 2013. Available from: https://api.semanticscholar.org/CorpusID:34575889 [Accessed: January 15, 2023]

[20] Scott RB. Historical review of legislative and national initiatives for sickle cell disease. The American Journal of Pediatric Hematology/Oncology. 1983;**5**(4):346-351. DOI: 10.1097/00043426-198324000-00006

[21] Sundd P, Gladwin MT, Novelli EM. Pathophysiology of sickle cell disease. Annual Review of Pathology. 2019;**14**:263-292. DOI: 10.1146/annurev-pathmechdis-012418-012838 Epub 2018 Oct 17

[22] Koch J. Robert Guthrie--the PKU Story: Crusade against Mental Retardation. California, USA: Hope Publishing House; 1997

[23] Association of Public Health, Laboratories Centers for Disease, Control Prevention. Hemoglobinopathies: Current Practices for Screening, Confirmation and Follow-up. 2015. Available from: https://stacks.cdc.gov/view/cdc/42387 [Accessed: March 23, 2022]

[24] Thuret I, Sarles J, Merono F, Suzineau E, Collomb J, Lena-Russo D, et al. Neonatal screening for sickle cell disease in France: Evaluation of the selective process. Journal of Clinical Pathology. 2010;**63**(6):548-551. DOI: 10.1136/jcp.2009.068874

[25] Okwi AL, Byarugaba W, Parkes A, Ocaido M. The reliability of sickling and solubility tests and peripheral blood film method for sickle cell disease screening at district health centers in Uganda. Clinics in Mother and Child Health. 2010;**7**(1):3

[26] de Haan K, Ceylan Koydemir H, Rivenson Y, Tseng D, Van Dyne E, Bakic L, et al. Automated screening of sickle cells using a smartphone-based microscope and deep learning. NPJ Digital Medicine. 2020;**3**:76

[27] Frommel C. Newborn screening for sickle cell disease and other Hemoglobinopathies: A short review on classical laboratory methods-isoelectric focusing, HPLC, and capillary electrophoresis. International Journal of Neonatal Screening. 2018;**4**(4):39

[28] Steele C, Sinski A, Asibey J, Hardy-Dessources M-D, Elana G, Brennan C, et al. Point-of-care screening for sickle cell disease in low-resource settings: A multi-center evaluation of HemoTypeSC, a novel rapid test. American Journal of Hematology. 2019;**94**(1):39-45

[29] Hernandez AG, Kiyaga C, Howard TA, Ssewanyana I, Ndeezi G, Aceng JR, et al. Trends in sickle cell trait and disease screening in the Republic of Uganda, 2014-2019. Tropical Medicine & International Health. 2021;**26**(1):23-32

[30] Ambrose EE, Smart LR, Charles M, Hernandez AG, Latham T, Hokororo A, et al. Surveillance for sickle cell disease, United Republic of Tanzania. Bulletin of the World Health Organization. 2020;**98**(12):859-868

[31] Nnodu O, Madu A, Chianumba R, Isa HA, Olanrewaju I, Osagie S, et al. Establishing a database for sickle cell disease patient mapping and survival tracking: The sickle pan-african research consortium Nigeria example. Frontiers in Genetics. 2022;**13**:1041462

[32] Alvarez OA, Hustace T, Voltaire M, Mantero A, Liberus U, Saint FR. Newborn screening for sickle cell disease using point-of-care testing in low-income setting. Pediatrics. 2019;**144**(4):e20184105

[33] Jain DL, Sarathi V, Upadhye D, Gulhane R, Nadkarni AH, Ghosh K, et al. Newborn screening shows a high incidence of sickle cell anemia in Central India. Hemoglobin. 2012;**36**(4):316-322

[34] Christopher HH, Burns A, Joscphat E, Saul S, Mgaya J, Makani J, et al. Evaluation of Newborns screening laboratory tests for sickle cell disease and other Haemoglobinopathies in Tanzania. Blood. 2019;**134**:4817

[35] Kanter J. Point-of-care testing in sickle cell disease. In: Sickle Cell Disease - Pain and Common Chronic Complications: London, United Kingdom: Intechopen Book Series. Editor B.P.D. Inusa; 2016

[36] Unger KK, Skudas R, Schulte MM. Particle packed columns and monolithic columns in high-performance liquid chromatography-comparison and critical appraisal. Journal of Chromatography A. 2008;**1184**(1):393-415

[37] Kutlar F, Kutlar A, Huisman TH. Separation of normal and abnormal hemoglobin chains by reversed-phase high-performance liquid chromatography. Journal of Chromatography. 1986;**357**(1):147-153

[38] Ndeezi G, Kiyaga C, Hernandez AG, Munube D, Howard TA, Ssewanyana I, et al. Burden of sickle cell trait and disease in the Uganda sickle surveillance study (US3): A cross-sectional study. The Lancet Global Health. 2016;**4**(3):e195-e200

[39] Arishi WA, Alhadrami HA, Zourob M. Techniques for the detection of sickle cell disease: A review. Micromachines. 2021;**12**(5):3-14

[40] Chindima N, Nkhoma P, Sinkala M, Zulu M, Kafita D, Simakando M, et al. The use of dried blood spots: A potential tool for the introduction of a neonatal screening program for sickle cell Anemia in Zambia. International Journal of Applied & Basic Medical Research. 2018;**8**(1):30-32

[41] Yue L, Lin M, Chen JT, Zhan XF, Zhong DS, Monte-Nguba SM, et al. Rapid screening for sickle cell disease by polymerase chain reaction-high resolution melting analysis. Molecular Medicine Reports. 2014;**9**(6):2479-2484

[42] Waterfall CM, Cobb BD. Single tube genotyping of sickle cell anaemia using PCR-based SNP analysis. Nucleic Acids Research. 2001;**29**(23):E119

[43] Newton CR, Graham A, Heptinstall LE, Powell SJ, Summers C, Kalsheker N, et al. Analysis of any point mutation in DNA. The amplification refractory mutation system (ARMS). Nucleic Acids Research. 1989;**17**(7):2503-2516

[44] Wilson JT, Milner PF, Summer ME, Nallaseth FS, Fadel HE, Reindollar RH, et al. Use of restriction endonucleases for mapping the allele for beta s-globin. Proceedings of the National Academy of Sciences of the United States of America. 1982;**79**(11):3628-3631

[45] Tripathi GR. A simplified and cheapest method for the diagnosis of sickle cell using whole blood PCR and RFLP in Nepal. Tribhuvan University Journal. 2016;**30**(2):57-64

[46] Ngole M, Race V, Mbayabo G, Lumbala P, Songo C, Lukusa PT, et al. DNA testing for sickle cell anemia in Africa: Implementation choices for the Democratic Republic of Congo. Journal of Clinical Laboratory Analysis. 2022;**36**(5):e24398

[47] Heather JM, Chain B. The sequence of sequencers: The history of sequencing DNA. Genomics. 2016;**107**(1):1-8

[48] Christopher H, Burns A, Josephat E, Makani J, Schuh A, Nkya S. Using DNA testing for the precise, definite, and low-cost diagnosis of sickle cell disease and other Haemoglobinopathies: Findings from Tanzania. BMC Genomics. 2021;**22**(1):902

[49] Adegoke SA, Oladimeji OI, Akinlosotu MA, Akinwumi AI, Matthew KA. HemoTypeSC point-of-care testing shows high sensitivity with alkaline cellulose acetate hemoglobin electrophoresis for screening hemoglobin SS and SC genotypes. Hematology, Transfusion and Cell Therapy. 2022;**44**(3):341-345

[50] Kettler H, White K, Hawkes SJ, Research UNWBWSPf, Training in Tropical D. Mapping the Landscape of Diagnostics for Sexually Transmitted Infections: Key Findings and Recommendations/Hannah Kettler, Karen White, Sarah Hawkes. Geneva: World Health Organization; 2004

[51] Land KJ, Boeras DI, Chen XS, Ramsay AR, Peeling RW. REASSURED diagnostics to inform disease control strategies, strengthen health systems and improve patient outcomes. Nature Microbiology. 2019;**4**(1):46-54

[52] Bond M, Hunt B, Flynn B, Huhtinen P, Ware R, Richards-Kortum R. Towards a point-of-care strip test to diagnose sickle cell anemia. PLoS One. 2017;**12**(5):e0177732

[53] Nnodu OE, Sopekan A, Nnebe-Agumadu U, Ohiaeri C, Adeniran A, Shedul G, et al. Implementing newborn screening for sickle cell disease as part of immunisation programmes in Nigeria: A feasibility study. The Lancet Haematology. 2020;**7**(7):e534-ee40

[54] Segbena AY, Guindo A, Buono R, Kueviakoe I, Diallo DA, Guernec G, et al. Diagnostic accuracy in field conditions of the sickle SCAN® rapid test for sickle cell disease among children and adults in two west African settings: The DREPATEST study. BMC Hematology. 2018;**18**(1):1-10

[55] Kanter J, Telen MJ, Hoppe C, Roberts CL, Kim JS, Yang X. Validation of a novel point of care testing device

for sickle cell disease. BMC Medicine. 2015;**13**(1):225

[56] Quinn CT, Paniagua MC, DiNello RK, Panchal A, Geisberg M. A rapid, inexpensive and disposable point-of-care blood test for sickle cell disease using novel, highly specific monoclonal antibodies. British journal of haematology. 2016;**175**(4):724-732

[57] Nnodu O, Isa H, Nwegbu M, Ohiaeri C, Adegoke S, Chianumba R, et al. HemoTypeSC, a low-cost point-of-care testing device for sickle cell disease: Promises and challenges. Blood Cells, Molecules, and Diseases. 2019;**78**:22-28

[58] Dexter D, McGann PT. Saving lives through early diagnosis: The promise and role of point of care testing for sickle cell disease. British Journal of Haematology. 2022;**196**(1):63-69

[59] Hasan MN, Fraiwan A, An R, Alapan Y, Ung R, Akkus A, et al. Paper based microchip electrophoresis for point-of-care hemoglobin testing. The Analyst. 2020;**145**(7):2525-2542

[60] Shrivas S, Patel M, Kumar R, Gwal A, Uikey R, Tiwari SK, et al. Evaluation of microchip-based point-of-care device "gazelle" for diagnosis of sickle cell disease in India. Frontiers in Medicine. 2021;**8**:1858

[61] Mukherjee MB, Colah RB, Mehta PR, Shinde N, Jain D, Desai S, et al. Multicenter evaluation of HemoTypeSC as a point-of-care sickle cell disease rapid diagnostic test for newborns and adults across India. American Journal of Clinical Pathology. 2020;**153**(1):82-87

[62] Makani J, Cox SE, Soka D, Komba AN, Oruo J, Mwamtemi H, et al. Mortality in sickle cell anemia in Africa: A prospective cohort study in Tanzania. PLoS One. 2011;**6**(2):e14699

[63] Smart LR, Ambrose EE, Raphael KC, Hokororo A, Kamugisha E, Tyburski EA, et al. Simultaneous point-of-care detection of anemia and sickle cell disease in Tanzania: The RAPID study. Annals of Hematology. 2018;**97**(2):239-246

[64] Alapan Y, Fraiwan A, Kucukal E, Hasan MN, Ung R, Kim M, et al. Emerging point-of-care technologies for sickle cell disease screening and monitoring. Expert Review of Medical Devices. 2016;**13**(12):1073-1093

[65] Yang X, Kanter J, Piety NZ, Benton M, Vignes SM, Shevkoplyas SS. A simple, rapid, low-cost test for the diagnosis of sickle cell disease using a paper-based hemoglobin solubility assay. Blood. 2012;**120**(21):245

[66] Piety NZ, George A, Serrano S, Lanzi MR, Patel PR, Noli MP, et al. Initial clinical validation of a rapid, low-cost, paper-based diagnostic test for sickle cell Anemia As a tool to facilitate Newborn screening in resource-limited settings. Blood. 2015;**126**(23):979

[67] Piety NZ, George A, Serrano S, Lanzi MR, Patel PR, Noli MP, et al. A paper-based test for screening newborns for sickle cell disease. Scientific Reports. 2017;7(1):1-8

[68] Piety NZ, Yang X, Kanter J, Vignes SM, George A, Shevkoplyas SS. Validation of a low-cost paper-based screening test for sickle cell Anemia. PLoS One. 2016;**11**(1):e0144901

[69] Kumar AA, Patton MR, Hennek JW, Lee SY, D'Alesio-Spina G, Yang X, et al. Density-based separation in multiphase systems provides a simple method to identify sickle cell disease. Proceedings of the National Academy of Sciences of the United States of America. 2014;**111**(41):14864-14869

[70] McGann PT, Hoppe C. The pressing need for point-of-care diagnostics for sickle cell disease: A review of current and future technologies. Blood Cells, Molecules, and Diseases. 2017;**67**:104-113

[71] Green NS, Mathur S, Kiguli S, Makani J, Fashakin V, LaRussa P, et al. Family, community, and health system considerations for reducing the burden of pediatric sickle cell disease in Uganda through newborn screening. Global. Pediatric Health. 2016;**3**:2333794X16637767

[72] Gibbons C, Geoghegan R, Conroy H, Lippacott S, O'Brien D, Lynam P, et al. Sickle cell disease: Time for a targeted neonatal screening programme. Irish Medical Journal. 2015;**108**(2):43-45

[73] Inusa BPD, Anie KA, Lamont A, Dogara LG, Ojo B, Ijei I, et al. Utilising the 'Getting to outcomes(®)' framework in community engagement for development and implementation of sickle cell disease Newborn screening in Kaduna state, Nigeria. International Journal of Neonatal Screening. 2018;**4**(4):33

[74] Anie KA, Treadwell MJ, Grant AM, Dennis-Antwi JA, Asafo MK, Lamptey ME, et al. Community engagement to inform the development of a sickle cell counselor training and certification program in Ghana. Journal of Community Genetics. 2016;7(3):195-202

[75] Mayo-Gamble TL, Murry VM, Cunningham-Erves J, Cronin RM, Lari N, Gorden A, et al. Engaging individuals with sickle cell disease in patient-Centered outcomes research: A community health ambassador training model A1. Journal of Health Care for the Poor and Underserved. 2020;**31**(1):353-369 PBJohns Hopkins University Press SN - 1548-6869 UR. Available from: https://musejhuedu/pub/1/article/747793

[76] Hines J, Mitchell MJ, Crosby LE, Johnson A, Valenzuela JM, Kalinyak K, et al. Engaging patients with sickle cell disease and their families in disease education, research, and community awareness. Journal of Prevention & Intervention in the Community. 2011;**39**(3):256-272

[77] Segbefia CI, Goka B, Welbeck J, Amegan-Aho K, Dwuma-Badu D, Rao S, et al. Implementing newborn screening for sickle cell disease in Korle Bu teaching hospital, Accra: Results and lessons learned. Pediatric Blood & Cancer. 2021;**68**(7):e29068

[78] Smart LR, Hernandez AG, Ware RE. Sickle cell disease: Translating clinical care to low-resource countries through international research collaborations. Seminars in Hematology. 2018;**55**(2):102-112

[79] Saint Fleur R, Archer N, Hustace T, Louis RJ, Bellevue R, Gautier J, et al. Capacity building and networking to make newborn screening for sickle cell disease a reality in Haiti. Blood Advances. 2018;**2**(Suppl 1):54-55

[80] McGann PT, Ferris MG, Ramamurthy U, Santos B, de Oliveira V, Bernardino L, et al. A prospective newborn screening and treatment program for sickle cell anemia in Luanda, Angola. American Journal of Hematology. 2013;**88**(12):984-989

[81] Treadwell MJ, Anie KA, Grant AM, Ofori-Acquah SF, Ohene-Frempong K. Using formative research to develop a counselor training program for newborn screening in Ghana. Journal of Genetic Counseling. 2015;**24**(2):267-277

[82] Ohene-Frempong K, Oduro J, Tetteh H, Nkrumah F. Screening newborns for sickle cell disease in Ghana. Pediatrics. 2008;**121**(Supplement_2):S120-S1S1

[83] Bukini D, Nkya S, McCurdy S, Mbekenga C, Manji K, Parker M, et al. Perspectives on building sustainable Newborn screening programs for sickle cell disease: Experience from Tanzania. International Journal of Neonatal Screening. 2021;7(1):14

[84] Streetly A. Screening infants for sickle cell disease in sub-Saharan Africa: Starting the journey to a sustainable model in primary care. The Lancet Haematology. 2020;7(7):e503-e5e4

Chapter 6

The Quality of Life of Children with Sickle Cell Disease (SCD)

Sampson Weytey

Abstract

Sickle cell disease (SCD) is known to be a major genetic condition that affects the populations of almost all the nations of the world, especially the African continent. Evidently, the trait of SCD has been said to have its roots in the soil of Africa, with an estimated prevalence rate between 10% and 40% among the entire population and among 300,000 children worldwide. SCD among children born in Africa has been estimated to have a prevalence rate of 75–85% and a mortality rate of 50–80% among children under 5 years. SCD is an inherited disorder in which there is a gene mutation that results in the abnormal sickle-shaped formation of the red blood cell (RBC) responsible for transporting oxygen throughout the body. The RBC, therefore, becomes harder, making it difficult to pass through smaller blood vessels, hence obstructing adequate blood flow and oxygen supply to the body cells and tissues. There are more devastating complications associated with SCD that have been linked with children than with adults, which include dactylitis and hand-foot syndrome, infections. SCD-related challenges have been well-documented, and studies have shown that the presence of these difficulties impacts daily living and subsequently, health-related quality of life (HRQOL) right from childhood. Most children in low- and middle-income countries (LMICs) are thought to pass away before reaching adulthood, with over 500 children with SCD dying each day due to inadequate access to appropriate treatment. Therefore, this chapter attempts to provide a thorough overview of the quality of life of children with SCD.

Keywords: quality of life, sickle cell disease, genetic, red blood cell, children, Africa, susceptibility, infection

1. Introduction

Millions of people worldwide are currently affected by sickle cell disease (SCD), the most prevalent hereditary hematologic illness that accounted for approximately 305,000 births in 2010 [1]. It is estimated that 200,000 neonates are impacted by sickle cell disease annually worldwide [2]. In the US, 70,000–100,000 people have sickle cell disease (SCD), and 2000 newborns are diagnosed with the condition every year [3, 4]. One in 300–400 African American births has it recognized among them [5]. Serious morbidities and early mortality are risks for children with sickle cell disease [6]. The first 3 years of life have the highest death rate of 50–90% among infants born in Africa [7].

Sickle cell disease (SCD) is a hereditary hemoglobin illness characterized by heterogeneity that results in endothelial dysfunction, vaso-occlusion, and persistent hemolytic anemia [8]. Multiple organ damage is frequently the result of these physiological disturbances during infancy and childhood [9]. Hemoglobin SC illness, sickle β thalassemia, and homozygous hemoglobin S (HbSS) disease are the three most prevalent forms of sickle cell disease [9, 10]. Because of their similar severity, sickle cell anemia and HbSS illness are frequently referred to as one another [11]. Only two structural hemoglobin (Hb) variants—Hb S and Hb C—achieve high frequency in Africa, despite the fact that over 700 Hb variants have been found [3]. Homozygous SCD is the most prevalent subtype of SCD globally [12]. The β-globin S (βS) mutation, which codes for sickle cell hemoglobin (Hb S), is present in two copies in these [13]. There are other names for homozygous SCD, including sickle cell anemia, Hb SS, SS, SS illness, and sickle cell disease-SS [14]. A recent global mapping of the βS allele's distribution using precise georeferenced data shows a strong correlation with the historical distribution of Plasmodium falciparum malarial endemicity [15].

SCD is one of the most well-known congenital illnesses in the world today [11]. It originated in Africa and was carried to the United States by the restricted movement of slaves [16]. Sickle cell disease (SCD) affects up to 3% of births in certain regions of sub-Saharan Africa, where it is widespread [17]. The early-life mortality of 50–90% among infants born in Africa with SS illness is consistent with the generally held belief that this ailment is linked to extremely high child mortality [18].

The last several decades have seen a significant improvement in the survival rate of young children with sickle cell disease [19]. Preventive penicillin, successful immunizations against *Streptococcus pneumoniae* and *Haemophilus influenzae* type B, and newborn screening are thought to be primarily responsible for the notable decline in early childhood mortality [20]. The various pathogenic processes causing organ malfunction and sickle cell events have been better understood within the last three decades [14]. Effective interventional techniques have been identified in a series of clinical trials [21]. Interventions that increase survival, avoid complications, treat acute events, and lessen end-organ damage are all part of the care for individuals with sickle cell disease (SCD) [21, 22]. Due to the higher risk of acute sickling complications and unexpected mortality, surgery under general anesthesia is one of the specific scenarios or circumstances in which patients with sickle cell disease (SCD) require particular care [23].

2. History behind sickle cell disease

Studies reveal that the mutation responsible for sickle cell disease originated in Africa thousands of years ago as a defense against malaria, which has historically been a leading cause of death in that continent [7]. The lack of the spleen was the main discovery made during the autopsy of an executed runaway slave, which may have been the earliest modern mention of sickle cell disease [11]. African slaves in the US reportedly showed resistance to malaria but were more likely to get leg ulcers [9]. First documented in 1910 [17], the aberrant properties of the red blood cells gave rise to the name of the illness by Ernest E. Irons (1877–1959) who was an intern of Chicago cardiologist and medical professor James B. Herrick (1861–1954) [16]. American physician James B. Herrick initially reported the hereditary disorder known as sickle cell disease in 1910 [19]. Before the twentieth century, SCD was recognized in a few regions of Africa [11]. As sickle cell disease developed throughout time, it was referred to by several names in African tribal languages [6]. People in western Africa gave the illness unique names that conjured up images of sudden, excruciating episodes or death, or that alluded to children who would die and then reincarnate as their own siblings [11, 24].

The mutation has appeared at least three times independently in Africa, according to the DNA structure surrounding the β-globin locus of HbS [7]. These mutations are known as β-globin haplotypes and are named after the countries where they were initially identified: Senegal, Benin, and Central African Republic or Bantu [24]. The HbC characteristic is thought to be a relatively recent mutation that is restricted to West Africa [2]. It is found at high frequencies (>20%) in central Ghana and Burkina Faso, in only 2% of Nigerians, and is absent from East and Central Africa with the exception of those who are descended from West Africans [14]. Regarding the kind and location of α- and β-thalassemia genes in Africa, there is a paucity of information [11, 24, 25]. SCD is one of the most well-known congenital illnesses in the world today [24].

3. Epidemiological studies

Worldwide, some 300,000 babies are born with sickle cell disease (SCD) each year, and the SCD population is well-documented in nations, including the United States, the United Kingdom, and Jamaica [26]. However, as more than 75% of SCD cases are found in sub-Saharan Africa, the cohort of SCD patients makes up just 1% of all SCD cases worldwide [27]. It is evident that Africa has the highest SCD mortality rate as well as the largest prevalence [28]. The majority of sickle cell disease patients reside in Africa, where the condition is poorly understood [29]. It is well-known, nevertheless, that the disease manifests itself in Africa more severely than it does elsewhere in the world [30].

SCD patients who are children have a greater death rate [30]. According to reports, most of these youngsters pass away in their early years if treatment is not received early [30, 31]. Research conducted in Nigeria revealed death rates as high as 90% [31], although more recent projections indicate that this percentage has dropped and is more likely to reach 50% in 20 years' time [32]. Africa's death rate is comparable to that of the United States and the United Kingdom in the early 1960s [33]. Nonetheless, substantial mortality reductions have been attained with early diagnosis and thorough treatment [1]. According to recent data, increased survival rates have been reached [30]; in the USA, 85.6% of patients survive to age 18 [34], in Jamaica, 84% to age 16, and in the UK, 99.0% to age 16 [34, 35]. With a birth frequency of one in 2415 in metropolitan France, SCD has emerged as the most prevalent genetic disease in France [22]. A 1998 study conducted on around 56,000 hospital patients in Bahrain revealed that 24% of respondents carried the gene mutation that causes sickle cell illness, 18% of respondents had the sickle cell trait, and 2% of babies had the condition [11].

As a result, SCD is highly prevalent at birth in Africa [35]. SCD, which was previously uncommon, has been brought to South Africa *via* internal migration, primarily from West and Central Africa [36]. The World Health Organization (WHO) designated sickle cell disease (SCD) as a public health priority in 2006 due to the high birth prevalence of SCD and its associated impact [20]. While the life expectancy for SCD patients is currently estimated to be between 45 and 55 years old in high-income settings, most children in low- and middle-income countries (LMICs) are thought to pass away before reaching adulthood, with over 500 children with SCD dying each day due to inadequate access to appropriate treatment [2]. Current estimates indicate that 90% of SCD cases occur in LMICs and 90% of SCD-affected children in LMICs pass away before turning five, underscoring this glaring difference [12].

The sickle cell trait is common in Saudi Arabia, but it is more prevalent in the eastern province [37]. The trait is most prevalent among the tribal peoples of central India (southern Tamil Nadu and Kerala), with a smaller concentration in the south (southeastern Gujarat, Maharashtra, Madhya Pradesh, Chhattisgarh, and western Odisha) with trait frequencies as high as 40% reported [32]. The Asian haplotype is named after these regions because the DNA structure surrounding the β-globin locus is different from that of African peoples, indicating that this is the fourth distinct instance of the HbS mutation [1]. This haplotype is frequently linked to frequent α-thalassemia and high amounts of fetal hemoglobin, both of which have the ability to prevent sickling and improve the clinical course [5]. In India and the Arabian Gulf, sickle cell disease is primarily known as SS illness [8].

4. Clinical manifestations of SCD among children

SCD is essentially a multisystem condition that affects practically every organ system in the body, despite its origins being an aberration of the red blood cell [31]. The most frequent diseases or consequences that were documented were discomfort, priapism, avascular necrosis (AVN) of the hips and shoulders, and asthma [26]. Prior research on hemoglobinopathies suggests that in response to pain or AVN, parent reports of physical functioning, sleep, and rest decreased [37]. Almost all functioning and weariness scores in children were negatively impacted by sickle pain and asthma to higher amount [7]. The term "crises" refers to a variety of symptoms that can include leg ulcers, discomfort, fever, anemia, exacerbation of jaundice, and specific syndromes, including acute chest syndrome (ACS) and acute splenic sequestration (ASS), dactylitis and hand-foot syndrome, growth retardation, delayed sexual maturation, underweight, and increased susceptibility to infections [2]. Also, facial droop, hemiparesis, seizures, dysarthria, headaches, and/or aphasia are common presentation symptoms [23].

5. Pathophysiology of SCD

The pathogenesis of this disease is primarily caused by hemoglobin polymerization, which results in erythrocyte stiffness and vaso-occlusion [11]. However, the significance of hemolysis, chronic anemia, and vasculopathy has already been shown [12]. People with sickle cell disease (SCD) are not anemic at birth, but they acquire chronic hemolytic anemia throughout their lives due to the synthesis of adult hemoglobin [33]. Acute periods of hemoglobin decrease, or "anemic crises," may occur in between [4]. The cause of sickle hemoglobin (HbS) is a substitution at position six of the β-globin polypeptide chain between the amino acid valine and glutamic acid [7]. The β-globin gene on chromosome 6 has a single-base mutation in codon 6 that results in the replacement of the sequence "GAG" for "GTG" [11]. Red blood cells (RBCs) carrying HbS become less malleable and take on a "sickle" shape when deoxygenated due to the aberrant amino acid in the β-globin chain, forming lengthy insoluble polymers [16].

It was previously believed that the defective stiff sickle red blood cell blocking small blood vessels was the only cause of the clinical repercussions [38]. Nonetheless, there is mounting evidence that a number of intricate processes that are not exclusive to the RBC are responsible for the pathophysiology of the different clinical episodes, both acute and chronic [8]. These include changes in the red cell membrane that cause the cell to become less sensitive to oxidative stress, the concentration of HbS, and other hemoglobin variations, such as fetal hemoglobin (HbF), within the cell, which decreases the cell's capacity to polymerize [8] and modified membrane lipids that lead to enhanced stiffness [1]. Furthermore, to mediate vaso-occlusion within the macro- and microvasculature, adhesion molecules such as integrins (α4 β1), (αv β3), their receptors (VCAM-1, ICAM-4), and selectins interact with endothelial cells, RBC, and a variety of soluble proteins within the plasma, such as thrombospondin (from platelets) and von Willebrand factor from endothelial cells [12–16].

Ultimately, strong evidence supports the involvement of nitric oxide (NO) in sickle cell disease [17]. Basal vasodilator tone is strongly regulated by NO [21]. Moreover, it prevents cellular adhesion molecules from being expressed [18]. There is more hemoglobin in the plasma than haptoglobin can scavenge due to the increased hemolysis in sickle cell disease [13]. As a result, aberrant "cell-free" hemoglobin is produced, which circulates in plasma and reduces the concentration of NO by binding to and consuming it [19]. Vasoconstriction enhanced leukocyte, endothelial cell, and erythrocyte adhesiveness, and platelet aggregation are the outcomes of this [7].

6. Laboratory and diagnostic investigation of SCD

With variations in the percentage of two other hemoglobin, HbF and HbA2, in RBCs, the laboratory diagnosis of sickle cell disease (SCD) is predicated on the presence of HbS, and the lack of appreciable decreases in HbA [2]. Hemoglobin levels in the 6–8 g/dl range and a high reticulocyte count are found in individuals with hemoglobin S disease (HbS) [17]. This is because the bone marrow produces extra red blood cells to make up for the destroyed sickled cells [14]. In order to confirm the sickle phenotype (SS/AS/SC/Sβ-thalassemia), screening procedures commonly available include the sodium metabisulphite sickling test, sickle solubility tests, and confirmation testing utilizing electrophoresis and chromatography [22]. High-performance liquid chromatography (HPLC), isoelectric focusing (IEF), and hemoglobin electrophoresis are the three most employed assays [16]. DNA-based techniques accurately characterize the genotype [38], however, screening (sickling or solubility test) and confirmation of the sickle phenotype by gel electrophoresis, IEF, or HPLC are typically required for diagnosis for clinical purposes [12].

7. Complications of SCD

The genetic hemoglobin anomaly that causes sickling of red blood cells, anemia, and problems from vaso-occlusion is known as sickle cell disease (SCD) [29]. In children, SCD can frequently result in excruciating pain and potentially fatal consequences affecting several organ systems [15]. Many millions of disability-adjusted life years are thought to be lost annually as a result of SCD, especially in poor nations [39]. The health impact of hemoglobinopathies alone is equivalent to that of major illnesses and communicable disorders [40]. According to reports, 14% of kids with SS-SCD may be functionally asplenic at 6 months of age [19]. This percentage then appears to rise over time, with affected pediatric patients being impacted at 1 year, 58% at 2 years, 78% at 3 years, and 94% at 5 years [8]. In addition to arterial endothelial damage and chronic hemolysis, sickle cell disease (SCD) raises the risk of acute and long-term organ system damage [28]. The majority of organs, including the brain, kidneys, lungs, bones, and cardiovascular system, gradually deteriorate as a result of repeated bouts of vaso-occlusion and inflammation [12].

The development of cerebrovascular illness and cognitive impairment is one of the primary issues associated with sickle cell disease in children [12]. Fever, dactylitis, and splenic sequestration are common problems in infants [29]. It has been documented that encapsulated organism infections, such as *Streptococcus pneumonia*, can affect children with sickle cell disease (SCD) [2]. This increased severity of sickle cell disease is a result of these viral illnesses [12]. In the past, 11% of people with SCD had experienced an ischemic or hemorrhagic stroke before turning 20 years [33]. Also, facial droop, hemiparesis, seizures, dysarthria, headaches, and or aphasia are common presenting complications [23]. In patients with sickle cell disease (SCD), acute chest syndrome (ACS) is the primary cause of death and the second most frequent cause of hospitalization [2].

Sickle cell disease, or hemoglobin S homozygosis, is the most frequent genotype and presents with the most severe clinical presentation of SCDs, even though other genotypes result in a lower life expectancy [6]. Patients with SCD have a higher death rate and a lower survival rate, according to several research [12–15]. Acute splenic sequestration and infections are the main causes of death before the age of 10 [30]. From the first year of life onward, acute complications and organ dysfunction are linked to significant morbidity in sickle cell anemia [38]. The USA, UK, and Jamaica have high rates of infection-related mortality, acute splenic sequestration, and acute chest syndrome [11, 24–28], with the largest incidence occurring in children aged one to three [38]. Infections, ACS, ASS, and aplastic crises are the leading causes of death in the United States, the United Kingdom, and Jamaica [24].

8. Various questionnaires used in assessing the health-related quality of life (HRQOL) of children with SCD

Evaluating the quality of life of children affected by sickle cell disease is essential [19]. This is done to comprehend their overall health, pinpoint areas in which they might require assistance, and customize interventions aimed at enhancing their quality of life [40]. While there are several methods and questionnaires available for assessing the quality of life of children with sickle cell disease (SCD), the most widely used ones are the Patient-Reported Outcomes Measurement Information System (PROMIS), the Pediatric Quality of Life Sickle Cell Disease Module (PedsQL SCD), Child Health Questionnaire, and Pediatric Quality of Life Inventory (PedsQL) 4.0 Generic Core Scales [41]. These questionnaires are used to evaluate juvenile sickle cell disease patients' quality of life [40]. They address a number of domains, including pain, exhaustion, worry, despair, physical capabilities, relationships with peers, sleep difficulties, and pain interference [42, 43].

9. Quality of life of children with SCD

SCD-related challenges have been well-documented, with studies showing that the presence of these difficulties impacts daily living and subsequently, health-related quality of life (HRQOL) of children [13]. An individual's overall assessment of the social, psychological, and physical facets of their existence is represented by the multi-faceted concept of quality of life (QOL) [5, 6]. It is a subjective rating that functions as a broad gauge of well-being that takes into account a variety of functional aspects [9]. Children with sickle cell disease (SCD) may be more susceptible to low quality of life since they are already at risk for a wide range of morbidities that affect many aspects of their functioning [5]. By keeping an eye on the health-related quality of life of children with sickle cell disease (SCD), one can gain a better knowledge of health status variations, identify potential SCD-related issues, and assess the need for therapeutic care [8]. Overall health-related quality of life and all of its subdomains are viewed by parents and children with SCD as being lower than it has been reported among healthy children [6]. As a result, effective therapeutic initiatives to enhance quality of life may signify significant advancements in the medical care of kids with SCD [10].

The majority of newborns diagnosed with sickle cell disease (SCD) during newborn screening are directed to their nearby hemoglobinopathy clinic for consistent monitoring [44]. Families may find it challenging to make their first appointment with the pediatric hematologist, especially if no family members have had SCD in the past [7]. Although the high quantity of fetal hemoglobin in infancy is usually protective, there are perhaps several difficulties that newborns with sickle cell disease face [28]. Disease-related issues have the potential to have a long-term detrimental influence on HRQL since children and adolescents are going through important periods in their physical, cognitive, and social-emotional development [12]. For instance, compared to their peers, children with SCD who experienced frequent pain reported missing up to 8 weeks of school and participating in fewer sports and other extracurricular activities [8]. Also, about 60% of teenagers in a different study stated that difficulties associated with their sickness, such as discomfort, infection, pneumonia, and subsequent hospital stays, affect their ability to perform academically [15, 16]. Illness-related chronic absenteeism affects social functioning and, consequently, HRQL [17, 18]. Furthermore, a number of studies have shown that children with sickle cell disease (SCD) had worse quality of life and more depressed symptoms when their parents provided them with less assistance [12]. A child's well-being may be impacted by the psychological and emotional effects of SCD since they may also experience despair, anxiety, and social isolation [13].

10. Management and prevention of SCD

The most severe type of sickle cell disease (SCD), sickle cell anemia (HbSS), causes 95% of children to survive their first 10 years of life, according to several empirical studies [5–8]. It is possible that advancements in early survival have only caused the mortality load to shift to later childhood [15]. Literature reports that children with sickle cell anemia (HbSS) have a survival rate of just 85.6% (95% confidence interval [CI]: 73.4–97.8) at the age of 18 [34, 35]. A number of straightforward interventions, such as newborn screening and infection prevention with penicillin prophylaxis and polyvalent pneumococcal vaccination, have all but eliminated elevated mortality from sickle cell disease (SCD) in children under the age of five in North America [13]. The United Nations has recognized sickle cell disease (SCD) as a global public health concern due to its debilitating effect on red blood cells and high rates of morbidity and mortality among younger people [45]. The World Health Organization (WHO) with this regard has also recommended more than 50% of its member states to establish SCD control programs [23].

In the United States, the use of oral penicillin against SCD has significantly reduced its rate of mortality [25], and many high-income nations now mandate that SCD patients to receive both antipneumococcal vaccination and penicillin prophylaxis [22, 23]. A number of SCD problems can also be avoided with certain therapies, such as hydroxyurea (HU) and routine transfusions [19], while for acute complications, analgesics, antibiotics, and blood transfusions are frequently required [14–19]. Hydroxyurea (HU) has been shown to be beneficial on rates of acute chest syndrome (ACS), vaso-occlusive crisis (VOC), hospitalization, and death in both adult and pediatric clinical trials [28]. Furthermore, increasing knowledge is being gained regarding the effectiveness of hydroxycarbamide and blood transfusions in preventing these problems [12].

In high-resource nations, such as the United States, the morbidity and death rates for children with sickle cell disease (SCD) have significantly decreased as a result of early detection through newborn screening programs, prophylactic therapy, and comprehensive care programs that include hydroxyurea therapy and bone marrow transplantation [41]. Patients with SCD in Africa can benefit from many of these therapies in the same ways [42]. The SCD burden in Africa can be decreased by newborn screening for the disease and by forming alliances between high-resource nations and African nations to fund healthcare worker training, research, and knowledge exchange [43–45]. For children with sickle cell disease (SCD), screening and preventive interventions—such as immunization and infection prophylaxis—have greatly improved results [46]. Evidence-based treatments, such as transfusion and hydroxyurea, are crucial in stopping the advancement of some problems [47].

Additionally, by collaborating and educating primary care physicians and pediatric hematopathologists to provide SCD-specific healthcare management, problems related to the disease can be reduced [48]. In order to lessen the impact of sickle cell disease (SCD) in the African region, the WHO Africa has recommended a number of public health interventions [48, 49]. These include raising awareness of the disease, preventing it, detecting it early, and improving the care given to affected individuals by providing efficient clinical, laboratory, diagnostic, and imaging facilities that are tailored to various levels of the healthcare system [50, 51]. Also, screening newborns, educating healthcare professionals, creating treatment protocols, offering genetic counseling, patient support groups, advocacy, and research are all recommended [51].

11. Conclusion

It is well-recognized that sickle cell disease (SCD) is a serious genetic ailment that affects people worldwide, mostly on the African continent. This condition has an estimated frequency rate of 10–40% across the total population and among 300,000 children worldwide. The trait of SCD is said to have originated in Africa and was carried to the United States by the restricted movement of slaves. According to empirical studies over the years, the prevalence of SCD among children born in Africa is 75–85%, and the mortality rate is 50–80% for children under five. Also, it is well-documented in nations including the United States, the United Kingdom, Jamaica, Saudi Arabia, and India. Many millions of disability-adjusted life years are thought to be lost annually as a result of SCD, especially in poor nations. A gene mutation causes the sickle-shaped development of red blood cells (RBCs), which are essential for carrying oxygen throughout the body. As a result, the RBC hardens and becomes more difficult to squeeze through tiny blood vessels, preventing the body's cells and tissues from receiving enough blood flow and oxygen.

Aplastic crisis, vaso-occlusive events, splenic sequestration, infections, underweight, delayed sexual maturation, dactylitis and hand-foot syndrome, growth retardation, and infections are just a few of the debilitating consequences of sickle cell disease (SCD) that have been linked to children. Research indicates that these issues have an impact on day-to-day functioning and, in turn, health-related quality of life (HRQOL) of children affected by it. About 60% of teenagers in different studies have stated that difficulties associated with their sickness, such as discomfort, infection, pneumonia, and subsequent hospital stays, affect their ability to perform academically. For clinical purposes, diagnosis usually requires screening (sickling or solubility test) and confirmation of the sickle phenotype by gel electrophoresis, IEF, or HPLC. High fluid intake, folic acid supplementation, high doses of immunizations and antibiotics, pain management, and infection prevention may all be beneficial for those with sickle cell disease.

Acknowledgements

Extending sincere gratitude to all authors and publishers of the books and articles used as references in this research work. Good wishes also to all who will find this review material useful in their specific field of study. Many appreciation and gratitude to the sponsors and funders of this research work. God bless. Thank you.

Conflict of interest

The author declares no conflict of interest.

Appendix and nomenclature

ACS	acute chest syndrome
ASS	acute splenic sequestration
AVN	avascular necrosis
HbF	fetus hemoglobin
Hb	hemoglobin
HRQoL	health-related quality of life
HU	hydroxyurea
IEF	isoelectric focusing
QoL	quality of life
NO	nitric oxide
PedsQL	Pediatric Quality of Life Inventory
PROMIS	Patient-reported Outcomes Measurement Information System
SCD	sickle cell disease
VOC	vaso-occlusive crisis
WHO	World Health Organization
HPLC	high-performance liquid chromatography

Author details

Sampson Weytey
Valley View University, Accra, Ghana

*Address all correspondence to: sampsonweytey@gmail.com

References

[1] McGann PT. Time to invest in sickle cell anemia as a global health priority. Pediatrics. 2016;**137**:e20160348. DOI: 10.1542/peds.2016-0348

[2] Kavanagh PL, Sprinz PG, Vinci SR, Bauchner H, Wang CJ. Management of children with sickle cell disease: A comprehensive review of the literature. Pediatrics. 2011;**128**(6):e1552-e1574. DOI: 10.1542/peds.2010-3686

[3] Diallo D, Tchernia G. Sickle cell disease in Africa. Current Opinion in Hematology. 2002;**9**(2):111-116. Available from: https://journals.lww.com/co-hematology/abstract/2002/03000/sickle_cell_disease_in_africa.5.aspx

[4] Ballas SK, Gupta K, Adams-Graves P. Sickle cell pain: A critical reappraisal. Blood. 2012;**120**:3647-3656. DOI: 10.1182/blood-2012-04-383430

[5] Wang CJ, Kavanagh PL, Little AA, Holliman JB, Sprinz PG. Quality-of-care indicators for children with sickle cell disease. Pediatrics. 2011;**128**(3):484-493. DOI: 10.1542/peds.2010-1791

[6] Makani J, Ofori-Acquah SF, Nnodu O, Wonkam A, Ohene-Frempong K. Sickle cell disease: New opportunities and challenges in Africa. Scientific World Journal. 2013;**2013**:193252. DOI: 10.1155/2013/193252

[7] Noronha SA, Sadreameli SC, Strouse JJ. Management of sickle cell disease in children. Southern Medical Journal. 2016;**109**(9):495-502. DOI: 10.14423/SMJ.0000000000000523

[8] Rees DC, Williams TN, Gladwin MT. Sickle-cell disease. The Lancet. 2010;**376**(9757):2018-2031. DOI: 10.1016/S0140-6736(10)61029-X

[9] Grosse SD, Odame I, Atrash HK, Amendah DD, Piel FB, Williams TN. Sickle cell disease in Africa: A neglected cause of early childhood mortality. American Journal of Preventive Medicine. 2011;**41**(6):S398-S405. DOI: 10.1016/j.amepre.2011.09.013

[10] Martins A, Galvão D, Emilia M, Nascimento EM, Soares E. Self-care for the treatment of leg ulcers in sickle cell anemia: Nursing guidelines. Escola Anna Nery. 2013;**17**(4):755-763. DOI: 10.5935/1414-8145.20130021

[11] Quinn CT, Rogers ZR, McCavit TL, Buchanan GR. Improved survival of children and adolescents with sickle cell disease. Blood, The Journal of the American Society of Hematology. 2010;**115**(17):3447-3452. DOI: 10.1182/blood-2009-07-233700

[12] Dampier C, Lieff S, LeBeau P, Rhee S, McMurray M, Rogers Z, et al. Health-related quality of life in children with sickle cell disease: A report from the comprehensive sickle cell centers clinical trial consortium. Pediatric Blood and Cancer. 2010;**55**(3):485-494. DOI: 10.1002/pbc.22497

[13] Noronha SA, Lanzkron S. Health Care Maintenance and Management of Chronic Complications of Sickle Cell Disease: A Pocket Guide for the Clinician. Washington, DC: American Society of Hematology; 2014. DOI: 10.1182/bloodadvances.2019000916

[14] Creary SE, Strouse JJ. Hydroxyurea and Transfusion Therapy for the Treatment of Sickle Cell Disease: A Pocket Guide for the Clinician. Washington, DC: American Society of Hematology; 2014. DOI: 10.1002/cpt.2028

[15] Aygun B, Mortier NA, Smeltzer MP, et al. Hydroxyurea treatment decreases glomerular hyperfiltration in children with sickle cell anemia. American Journal of Hematology. 2013;**88**:116-119. DOI: 10.1002/ajh.23365

[16] Almeida CB, Souza LE, Leonardo FC, et al. Acute hemolytic vascular inflammatory processes are prevented by nitric oxide replacement or a single dose of hydroxyurea. Blood. 2015;**126**:711-720. DOI: 10.1182/blood-2014-12-616250

[17] Yee MM, Jabbar SF, Osunkwo I, et al. Chronic kidney disease and albuminuria in children with sickle cell disease. Clinical Journal of the American Society of Nephrology. 2011;**6**:2628-2633. DOI: 10.2215/CJN.01600211

[18] Alvarez O, Miller ST, Wang WC, et al. Effect of hydroxyurea treatment on renal function parameters: Results from the multi-center placebo-controlled BABY HUG clinical trial for infants with sickle cell anemia. Pediatric Blood & Cancer. 2012;**59**:668-674. DOI: 10.1002/pbc.24100

[19] McCavit T, Desai P. Management of Acute Complications of Sickle Cell Disease: A Pocket Guide for the Clinician. Washington, DC: American Society of Hematology; 2014. Available from: https://www.ncbi.nlm.nih.gov/books/NBK566466/

[20] Wastnedge E, Waters D, Patel S, Morrison K, Goh MY, Adeloye D, et al. The global burden of sickle cell disease in children under five years of age: A systematic review and meta-analysis. Journal of Global Health. Dec 2018;**8**(2):021103. DOI: 10.7189/jogh.08.021103

[21] Manwani D, Frenette PS. Vaso-occlusion in sickle cell disease: Pathophysiology and novel targeted therapies. Blood. 2013;**122**:3892-3898. DOI: 10.1182/blood-2013-05-498311

[22] Dale JC, Cochran CJ, Roy L, Jernigan E, Buchanan GR. Health-related quality of life in children and adolescents with sickle cell disease. Journal of Pediatric Health Care. 2011;**25**(4):208-215. DOI: 10.1016/j.pedhc.2009.12.006

[23] Meier ER, Miller JL. Sickle cell disease in children. Drugs. 2012;**72**: 895-906. Available from: https://link.springer.com/article/10.2165/11632890-000000000-00000

[24] Fernandes AP, Januário JN, Cangussu CB, Macedo DL, Viana MB. Mortality of children with sickle cell disease: A population study. Jornal de Pediatria. 2010;**86**:279-284. DOI: 10.1590/S0021-75572010000400006

[25] Mulumba LL, Wilson L. Sickle cell disease among children in Africa: An integrative literature review and global recommendations. International Journal of Africa Nursing Sciences. 2015;**3**:56-64. DOI: 10.1016/j.ijans.2015.08.002

[26] US Department of Health and Human Services. Evidence-Based Management of Sickle Cell Disease: Expert Panel Report. 2014. Available from: https://www.nhlbi.nih.gov/sites/www.nhlbi.nih.gov/files/sickle-cell-disease-report.pdf

[27] Bartolucci P, Chaar V, Picot J, et al. Decreased sickle red blood cell adhesion to laminin by hydroxyurea is associated with inhibition of Lu/BCAM protein phosphorylation. Blood. 2010;**116**:2152-2159. DOI: 10.1182/blood-2009-12-257444

[28] Chaar V, Laurance S, Lapoumeroulie C, et al. Hydroxycarbamide decreases

sickle reticulocyte adhesion to resting endothelium by inhibiting endothelial lutheran/basal cell adhesion molecule (Lu/BCAM) through phosphodiesterase 4A activation. The Journal of Biological Chemistry. 2014;**289**:11512-11521. DOI: 10.1074/jbc.M113.506121

[29] Dowell D, Haegerich TM, Chou R. CDC guideline for prescribing opioids for chronic pain—United States, 2016. MMWR - Recommendations and Reports. 2016;**65**:1-49. DOI: 10.1001/jama.2016.1464

[30] Kassim AA, Galadanci NA, Pruthi S, et al. How I treat and manage strokes in sickle cell disease. Blood. 2015;**125**:3401-3410. DOI: 10.1182/blood-2014-09-551564

[31] DeBaun MR, Gordon M, McKinstry RC, et al. Controlled trial of transfusions for silent cerebral infarcts in sickle cell anemia. The New England Journal of Medicine. 2014;**371**:699-710. DOI: 10.1056/NEJMoa1401731

[32] Kawadler JM, Clayden JD, Clark CA, et al. Intelligence quotient in paediatric sickle cell disease: A systematic review and meta-analysis. Developmental Medicine and Child Neurology. 2016;**58**:672-679. DOI: 10.1111/dmcn.13113

[33] King AA, Strouse JJ, Rodeghier MJ, et al. Parent education and biologic factors influence on cognition in sickle cell anemia. American Journal of Hematology. 2014;**89**:162-167. DOI: 10.1002/ajh.23604

[34] Therrell BL Jr, Lloyd-Puryear MA, Eckman JR, et al. Newborn screening for sickle cell diseases in the United States: A review of data spanning 2 decades. Seminars in Perinatology. 2015;**39**:238-251. DOI: 10.1053/j.semperi.2015.03.008

[35] Hebson C, New T, Record E, et al. Elevated tricuspid regurgitant velocity as a marker for pulmonary hypertension in children with sickle cell disease: Less prevalent and predictive than previously thought? Journal of Pediatric Hematology/Oncology. 2015;**37**:134-139. DOI: 10.1097/MPH.0000000000000184

[36] Boulet SL, Yanni EA, Creary MS, Olney RS. Health status and healthcare use in a national sample of children with sickle cell disease. American Journal of Preventive Medicine. 2010;**38**(4):S528-S535. DOI: 10.1016/j.amepre.2010.01.003

[37] Piel FB, Hay SI, Gupta S, Weatherall DJ, Williams TN. Global burden of sickle cell anaemia in children under five, 2010-2050: Modelling based on demographics, excess mortality, and interventions. PLoS Medicine. 2013;**10**:e1001484. DOI: 10.1371/journal.pmed.1001484

[38] Chakravorty S, Williams TN. Sickle cell disease: A neglected chronic disease of increasing global health importance. Archives of Disease in Childhood. 2015;**100**:48-53. DOI: 10.1136/archdischild-2013-303773

[39] Munaretto V, Reggiani G, Munerol C, Maran E, Perdibon M, Frigo AC, et al. Quality of life in children, adolescents and young adults with sickle cell disease and their caregivers during standard of care and after bone marrow transplantation: A single center report. Blood. 2021;**138**:3032. DOI: 10.1182/blood-2021-151297

[40] Esham KS, Rodday AM, Smith HP, Noubary F, Weidner RA, Buchsbaum RJ, et al. Assessment of health-related quality of life among adults hospitalized with sickle cell disease vaso-occlusive crisis. Blood Advances. 2020;**4**(1):19-27. DOI: 10.1182/bloodadvances.2019000128

[41] Smyth M, Jacobson K. Pediatric Quality of Life Inventory^{TM} version 4.0 short form generic core scale across pediatric populations review data. Data in Brief. 2021;**39**:107599. DOI: 10.1016/j.dib.2021.107599

[42] Menezes AS, Len CA, Hilário MO, Terreri MT, Braga JA. Quality of life in patients with sickle cell disease. Revista Paulista de Pediatria. 2013;**31**:24-29. DOI: 10.1590/S0103-05822013000100005

[43] Weatherall D. The inherited disorders of haemoglobin: An increasingly neglected global health burden. The Indian Journal of Medical Research. 2011;**134**:493-497. Available from: https://pubmed.ncbi.nlm.nih.gov/22089613/

[44] de Castro L, Lobo C, Pinto JF, Nascimento EM, Moura PG, Cardoso GP, et al. The effect of hydroxcarbamide therapy on survival of children with sickle cell disease. British Journal of Haematology. 2013;**161**(6):852-860. DOI: 10.1111/bjh.12323

[45] Wang WC, Ware RE, Miller ST, Iyer RV, Casella JF, Minniti CP, et al. Hydroxycarbamide in very young children with sickle-cell anaemia: A multicentre, randomised, controlled trial (BABY HUG). The Lancet. 2011;**377**(9778):1663-1672. DOI: 10.1016/S0140-6736(11)60355-3

[46] Porter M. Rapid fire: Sickle cell disease. Emergency Medicine Clinics. 2018;**36**(3):567-576. Available from: https://www.emed.theclinics.com/article/S0733-8627(18)30025-7/fulltext

[47] Stokoe M, Zwicker HM, Forbes C, Abu-Saris NE, Fay-McClymont TB, Désiré N, et al. Health related quality of life in children with sickle cell disease: A systematic review and meta-analysis. Blood Reviews. 2022;**56**:100982. DOI: 10.1016/j.blre.2022.100982

[48] Sehlo MG, Kamfar HZ. Depression and quality of life in children with sickle cell disease: The effect of social support. BMC Psychiatry. 2015;**15**:1-8. Available from: https://link.springer.com/article/10.1186/s12888-015-0461-6

[49] Serjeant GR. The natural history of sickle cell disease. Cold Spring Harbor Perspectives in Medicine. 1 Oct 2013;**3**(10):a011783. DOI: 10.1101/cshperspect.a011783

[50] Grosse SD, Atrash HK, Odame I, Amendah D, Piel FB, Williams TN. The Jamaican historical experience of the impact of educational interventions on sickle cell disease child mortality. American Journal of Preventive Medicine. 2012;**42**(6):e101-e103. Available from: https://www.ajpmonline.org/article/S0749-3797(12)00175-4/fulltext

[51] Silva IV, Reis AF, Palaré MJ, Ferrao A, Rodrigues T, Morais A. Sickle cell disease in children: Chronic complications and search of predictive factors for adverse outcomes. European Journal of Haematology. 2015;**94**(2):157-161. DOI: 10.1111/ejh.12411